Amputations and Prostheses

This book is dedicated to the late Mr St John Dudley Buxton FRCS, the late Mr Leon Gillis FRCS and the late Mr R. Langdale Kelham FRCS, who pioneered this important field and made Roehampton an international centre of amputation surgery and prosthetics.

—— SECOND EDITION ——

Amputations and Prostheses

Miroslaw Vitali OBE, MD, FRCS

Formerly Principal Medical Officer,
Department of Health and Social Security Limb Fitting Centre,
Roehampton; Honorary Consultant, Queen Mary's Hospital,
Rochampton, and the Westminster Hospital, London;
Honorary Adviser in Prosthetics and Prosthetic Surgery,
Institute of Orthopaedics, Royal National Orthopaedic Hospital,
Stanmore, Middlesex

Kingsley P. Robinson MS, FRCS (Ed), FRCS

Director of Limb-Surgery Unit and Consultant Surgeon,
Queen Mary's Hospital, Roehampton;
Consultant Surgeon, Westminster Hospital, London

Brian G. Andrews FRCS, MB, BS, LRCP

Consultant Orthopaedic Surgeon,
Westminster Hospital and Queen Mary's Hospital, Roehampton;
Honorary Consultant, Department of Health and Social Security
Limb Fitting Centre, Roehampton;
Sub-Dean, Charing Cross and Westminster Medical School, London;
Member of the Court of Examiners,
Royal College of Surgeons of England

Edward E. Harris MA (Cantab), MRCS, LRCP

Formerly Deputy Medical Director,
Chailey Heritage Craft Schools and Hospitals;
Formerly Medical Officer,
Department of Health and Social Security
Limb Fitting Centre, Roehampton;
Formerly Staff Surgeon, Committee for
Prosthetic Research and Development,
National Academy of Sciences, Washington, USA

Robin G. Redhead MB, BS, MRCS, LRCP, PhD

Senior Medical Officer, Department of Health and Social Security
Limb Fitting Centre, Roehampton, London

Baillière Tindall London Philadelphia Toronto
Mexico City Sydney Tokyo Hong Kong

Baillière Tindall   1 St Anne's Road
W.B. Saunders   Eastbourne, East Sussex BN21 3UN, England

West Washington Square
Philadelphia, PA 19105, USA

1 Goldthorne Avenue
Toronto, Ontario M8Z 5T9, Canada

Apartado 26370 – Cedro 512
Mexico 4, DF Mexico

ABP Australia Ltd, 44–50 Waterloo Road
North Ryde, NSW 2113, Australia

Ichibancho Central Building, 22–1 Ichibancho
Chiyoda-ku, Tokyo 102, Japan

10/fl, Inter-Continental Plaza, 94 Granville Road
Tsim Sha Tsui East, Kowloon, Hong Kong

First published 1978
Second edition 1986

Typeset by Inforum Ltd, Portsmouth
Printed and bound in Great Britain by
Butler and Tanner Ltd, Frome and London

British Library Cataloguing in Publication Data

Amputations and prostheses.—2nd ed.
 1. Amputation   2. Artificial limbs
 I. Vitali, M.   II. Redhead, R.G.
 617'.58059   RD553

 ISBN 0–7020–0990–3

Contents

Preface

This second edition has been extensively revised. This is not only to reflect the changes made possible by technical advances in both surgery and external limb prosthetics but also to emphasize that amputation surgery and prosthetics are not separate entities and should be an integrated whole.

Miroslaw Vitali
Kingsley P Robinson
Brian G Andrews
Edward E Harris
Robin G Redhead

The basic principles of amputation surgery and external limb prosthetic design, within the limits of current techniques, are international. Custom, creed, climate, cost, available skills and materials give rise to regional variation but the general principles are the same worldwide and, for that reason, two chapters have been included on the fundamental basis of current practices.

While the authors hope that many experienced in amputation surgery and artificial limb replacement will read it with interest, the intention is to give those less experienced a clear guidance on procedures which will give a satisfactory amputation stump for prosthetic use. At each advocated level a specific surgical procedure is described that will give such a stump. Common variations used by some surgeons and comments on their advantages and disadvantages are also given.

Prosthetic design and mechanisms are largely illustrated from the practice in the United Kingdom but comparable materials and mechanisms are available and used in most countries.

We cannot hope to acknowledge all who have contributed to the advances. North America (the USA and Canada), Europe (Germany, France, Italy, Switzerland, Denmark, Sweden, Yugoslavia, Poland), and Asia (Japan, India and China) have all contributed, as have many other countries.

The authors, who now include Dr RG Redhead, senior medical officer at the Roehampton Limb-Fitting Centre, wish to acknowledge those who have helped them in the preparation of this second edition: Dr A Gregory Dean, who updated the chapter on Statistics; Dr Ian Fletcher, for revising the chapter on Upper-Limb Prosthetics and writing the chapter on Congenital Deformities; Miss Rosalind Ham and Mrs Penny Buttershaw for the chapter on Principles of Rehabilitation; Brigadier S Janikoun OBE FRCS; Mr George Kotas, medical illustrator; Mr N Babbage, consultant photographer, Bioengineering Centre, University College, London, for excellent photographic work; JE Hanger & Co. Ltd, CA Blatchford & Co., Vessa Ltd, and Hugh Steeper (Roehampton Ltd) for permission to use photographs and technical data of their products; and Miss Pat Young for editorial help and for keeping all of us under her firm controlling hand.

Lastly, the authors would wish to thank Dr Donald Acheson, chief medical officer, Department of Health and Social Security, for giving the book his official blessing; and Dr AW English, principal medical officer in charge of the Limb-Fitting Service, Department of Health and Social Security, for his continuing interest.

1

A Brief Historical Survey

Amputation is a destructive operation which removes but does not cure; but it can be constructive when it removes disability and disease to restore ability and ease. The dictum of Sir William Ferguson that 'Amputation is one of the meanest yet one of the greatest operations in Surgery; mean when resorted to where better could be done — great as the only step to give comfort in life' is as true today as when first written.

To restore function at most levels of amputation requires the use of an appliance or prosthesis which is attached to the body. This prosthesis may be simple in design and crude in appearance, such as a peg-leg or arm-hook. If nothing better is available these may be accepted by patients for their practical use. Through amputation the patient has lost not only part of his body but also part of his body image, so that to restore function involves psychological as well as physical replacement. He seeks a prosthesis which replaces the lost member in appearance, feel and movement: that is to say, an artificial limb. Prostheses currently in use usually resemble the lost limb in appearance but are normally of hard materials such as metal or wood so that they do not feel natural to the patient or to others. In many countries efforts are now being made to use methods of construction which will give some softness to touch.

Movement is an essential part of appearance and function and requires a source of power. External power has severe limitations in providing enough of either quantity or quality and is likely only to supplement power derived from the body rather than to replace it. The amputation stump and body, therefore, are the major, and usually the only, source of power for the operation of the prosthesis and need to be fashioned to join with it to give the best use if the prosthesis is to be an artificial limb.

This book is about the union of the stump and the prosthesis to form a single locomotor unit.

Neolithic man is known to have survived amputation and archaeologists claim that the remains of Neanderthal man show evidence that he lived after having lost a limb. Amputations among these primitive peoples were probably by accident, for punishment or during magic ritual rather than with surgical intent. There is no record of amputation in the Old Testament nor do the Egyptian medical papyri give any account of it. Although artificial limbs have been found on mummies with congenital or traumatic limb deficiencies, they are considered to be examples of the embalmer's art only and there is no evidence that they were ever used in life. In the Rig-veda of 1500 to 800 BC it is said that there is a reference to artificial limbs, but it is usually considered that the first account of amputation as a purposeful medical procedure is in the Hippocratic treatise *On Joints*, which has a modern ring about it for it is concerned with amputation in vascular gangrene. Indeed, surgical amputation in warfare, with which the condition is usually associated, does not seem to have been common until the use of gunpowder.

The early surgeon had knives and saws with which to amputate but lacked anaesthetics, tourniquets and ligatures. His enemies were shock, haemorrhage and sepsis. Mid-thigh and above-elbow amputations were rare because they were usually fatal. William Clowes (1588) is credited with the first known successful above-knee amputation. It must be doubted, however, whether this was indeed the first, for Paré in his *Œuvres* (1575) illustrates a complex prosthesis for the above-knee amputation. John Hunter said in about 1786 that 'an amputation below the knee in most cases would not kill by its haemorrhage'. The smaller bore of the vessels in the forearm and below the knee, combined with arteriospasm and surgical shock, would prevent fatal haemorrhage before the blood clotted. Hippocrates, who advocated amputation for vascular gangrene, advised that it should be through the ischaemic tissue at the joint below the boundaries of the blackening. He also described amputation by disarticulation at the knee.

Hippocrates also refers to the use of cautery for haemostasis and it has remained in use through the succeeding centuries to the present day. There are many references to the use of cautery in the ancient surgical treatises of Avicenna and Abulcasis, for example. It not only controlled haemorrhage from smaller vessels but was used by later surgeons for its antiputrefactive qualities; Peter Lowe (1597) preferred 'the ligature for haemorrhage when suppuration is not present; when it is, the cautery'. Even Paré used the cautery in gangrenous wounds and as late as 1924 Cullen was using cautery to control phagedenic gangrene.

The cautery would not control haemorrhage from major vessels; for this ligation was necessary. Celsus in the first century and Yperman in the thirteenth both used ligatures, although it is not recorded specifically that they used them in amputation. It was Ambroise Paré who reintroduced ligation for large vessels during amputation; this did not supplant the cautery for smaller vessels until the introduction of the tourniquet and anaesthetics. The surgeon worked without skilled aid. Two assistants restrained the patient, one plied him with pain-relieving drugs or drinks and a fourth handed the instruments. Speed was essential to lessen shock but became for many surgeons an objective in itself; Ferguson (1845) said that any surgeon should be able to amputate in 30 seconds and complete the procedure in three minutes. To tie ligatures in these circumstances without modern artery forceps must have been difficult. It is not surprising, therefore, that Guillemeau (1594), who was Paré's pupil and biographer, gave up ligation because of these difficulties.

The use of the tourniquet made ligation easier. Its invention is usually attributed to Morel (1674) during the siege of Besançon, but many earlier surgeons such as Botallus (1560) and Fabricus von Hilden used one or more tight bands round the limb, amputating below or between them, with the object of reducing pain and lessening bleeding. Later Petit (1718) used a compressive tourniquet and in 1873 Esmarch introduced the rubber bandage. A tourniquet is still part of the postoperative bedside equipment to stop any secondary haemorrhage.

Styptics such as alum, vitriol and turpentine were used to control oozing but their benefit, particularly that of oil of turpentine, may have been in their antiseptic properties. For if the patient survived the shock and haemorrhage of the operation he might be lucky to survive the subsequent sepsis. It is difficult to realize that surgeons seemed almost to glory in avoiding even normal social cleanliness in their professional work, so that it was even said that it was less dangerous for a patient to have his thigh amputated by gunfire than by a surgeon. Malgaigne (1842) reported a mortality of 62% in thigh amputations from nine Paris hospitals. Indeed, to have even a digit amputated was not without risk. This is not surprising when the description of Dupuytren operating is that 'he wore a dirty white apron, superfluously protecting a dirtier pair of trousers, a greasy threadbare coat and well-worn carpet shoes'. Pirogoff (1864) wrote of the sepsis in the surgical wards and of the few of the many thousands of amputees whom he knew to have survived; but Pirogoff, operating without gloves, suffered for 16 years from an intractable diarrhoea which only relented during periods of vacation. Bigelow's assistants at the Massachusetts General Hospital carried their sutures in the button-holes of their operation coats in the 1870s and as late as the 1880s assistants in some New York hospitals held the sutures in their mouths. This despite the writings of Thomson and Blackadder in the early years of the century that 'pouriture d'hôpital' was transferred from patient to patient only by soiled dressings. There were others whose standards would have been more acceptable in the present day. Monro (1752) reported on 99 amputations in Edinburgh Royal Infirmary with only eight deaths and in 1782 Alanson of Liverpool reported 35 without mortality. Among other surgeons who advocated cleanliness and had similar results were Maunoir (1825) of Geneva, Lister (1841) of London and Eve (1846) in Augusta.

The postoperative treatment of the wound changed with the centuries. The early hippocratic practice of amputating through devitalized tissue made it necessary for the wound to be left open so as to heal by granulation. When Celsus operated through viable tissue he divided the bone at a higher level than the soft tissues, thus allowing them to fall together over the bone. Ambroise Paré approximated the edges of the wound with adhesive strips, which Von Gersdorff also did at a later date, using an animal's bladder for cover in addition, and Brunschwig used a combination of sutures and bandaging. The method of

amputation was circular until Yonge and Lowdham (1679) introduced the flap amputation which made closure easier. The risk
of developing a haematoma led many surgeons to delay dressing
the wound for several hours. Liston had cold water compresses
applied to the wound every ten minutes for seven hours or
longer, until it developed a glazed appearance, before closing it
with adhesive tape. Primary closure was, however, often contraindicated by the presence of contamination, and many military
surgeons would agree with Stephen Smith (1862) when he wrote
'in the after treatment of the amputation . . . it is good practice
to leave the wounds open to heal by granulation'.

The advent of modern surgery, with the introduction of anaesthetics and later antiseptics and asepsis, enabled the surgeons to
develop techniques before the First World War which were very
similar to those in use today in that muscle flaps were used.
Unfortunately the surgeon's art then began to outstrip the limb-
maker's craft. Although that war saw the extended use of the
light metal limb, in the post-war years good amputation operations were revised to their detriment or abandoned to meet the
requirements of the limb-makers. The suturing of muscles over
the divided bone ends was abandoned and muscles were allowed
to retract in order to produce a 'conical' stump. The bulbous
end-bearing stumps produced by knee disarticulation and
Syme's amputation were taboo because they could not be introduced into a tube from above. It required the aftermath of a
Second World War to stimulate once again the study of amputations and prosthetics as a unity.

Prostheses themselves have a history as old as amputation.
There is a reference in the Rig-veda to artificial limbs, but the
earliest reference to amputation itself is usually considered to be
Herodotus (424 BC) who tells of Hegistratus of Elis, a seer who
was condemned to death by the Spartans. He was tethered by his
leg to await execution but escaped by amputating his foot himself
and travelling 30 miles to Tregea. At Zaccynthius he was again
captured by the Spartans who this time put him to death, but
recorded that he had been provided with a wooden foot. Simple
peg-legs made of wood are known to have been used in early
times from illustrations such as the mosaic in the cathedral of
Lescar in France; this shows one, used after an amputation by
disarticulation at the knee, which resembles one both described
and illustrated by Paré, as well as the 'Chelsea' peg used up to the
present day. The earliest surviving example of a prosthesis was
Roman, dated about 300 BC; made of bronze and wood, it can be
called an artificial limb as it was shaped to resemble the thigh,
knee and calf. Unfortunately it was lost with much else when the
Royal College of Surgeons' Museum was destroyed in an air raid.

The wooden peg – simple and cheap to make, stable in use and
easy to maintain – was the prosthesis of the peasants and poor
throughout the ages but did not satisfy the aesthetic needs of the
rich, who had servants to carry them over short distances and
horses for longer. The bearers of arms turned to their armourers

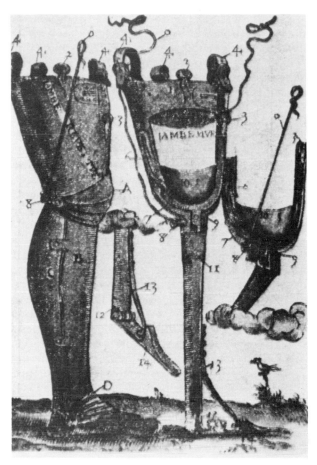

Fig 1.1 Artificial limbs designed by Ambroise Paré, primarily for wounded soldiers, and illustrated in his *Instrumenta Chirurgiae et Icones Anatomica* (1564)

to produce prostheses to resemble their armour. Many of these were functional as well as decorative, but were fashioned in iron and therefore heavy. One leg in the fine Stilbert collection in Florence has a rigid knee which is semi-flexed, suitable neither for standing nor for sitting but adequate for riding astride a charger. Paré devised and illustrated artificial legs made of iron which were of considerable complexity. Verduin (1696) produced the first artificial limb for below-knee amputees which had a leather socket and thigh corset with articulated side steels. It is not known when wooden artificial limbs other than simple legs were first introduced, but the simple wood 'clapper' limb was probably introduced by makers such as Grossmith who was working in London in 1750. Crowdero in Samuel Butler's *Hudibras* published in 1662 wears an oak peg. James Potts of London is said to have introduced the wooden leg in 1800. His limb showed great craftsmanship as well as ingenuity; the ankle and knee movements were coordinated by means of artificial tendons. Potts' most famous patron was the Marquis of Anglesey who lost his leg at Waterloo and whose name is still used for limbs made in this fashion.

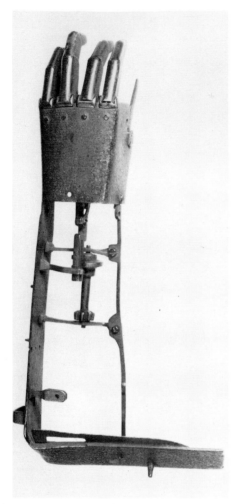

Fig 1.2   An iron artificial left hand and arm, dated about 1602. The thumb is fixed but all the fingers are movable. (*By courtesy of the Wellcome Trustees*)

The simple hook for the forearm amputation has been in use for many centuries, providing a useful tool for those earning a livelihood but wholly unacceptable aesthetically. Prostheses resembling the shape of a hand appeared early and showed considerable ingenuity in their construction. Pliny reports that Marius Sergius, who lost his right hand in the Second Punic War (218–202 BC), was fitted with an iron hand. The Alt-Ruppin hand, discovered in AD 1800 along the river Rhine and preserved in the Stilbert collection, is dated about AD 1400. It is made of iron and has a rigid thumb fixed in opposition and flexible fingers operating in pairs which were flexed passively, locking into position with a ratchet mechanism; it also has a movable wrist.

Perhaps the most famous user of an iron hand was a German knight, Gotz von Berlichingen, mentioned in a poem by Goethe, who lost his hand at the siege of Landshut (1509). Several versions of the iron hand which he used exist. The fingers of this hand also could be flexed passively by the other hand and locked into position by a ratchet. '*Le petit Lorraine*' is another iron hand described and illustrated by Ambroise Paré.

All these ingenious and elaborate hands are extremely heavy and of limited use, as they depend on the opposite hand for operation. It was not until 1818 that the prosthesis was given any power of prehension by harnessing the shoulder girdle muscles, a system devised by a Berlin dentist called Peter Ballif. This was for a forearm amputation only. The same principle was not applied to the above-elbow prosthesis until 1844 when a Dutchman, Van Peetersen, used it for elbow flexion. By 1855 the Comte de Beaufort was demonstrating an arm with elbow flexion activated by pressure of a lever against the chest and in 1867 he published an illustration of an operating harness which resembles the harness in use today.

Wars give impetus to the use of artificial devices to replace limb deficiencies. The Second World War was no exception but whereas real advance after other wars was slow, the Second World War was followed by a scientific and technological explosion leading to major changes in methods of amputation and design of prostheses throughout the world.

There have been research programmes since the First World War, but the programme organized in 1945 by the United States National Academy of Sciences, at the request of the Surgeon-General of the army, provided resources which not only promoted development domestically but also stimulated worldwide interest. The programme provided both fundamental research and development of an educational programme for physicians, remedial therapists and prosthetists.

The Committee on Prostheses, Braces and Technical Aids of the International Society for the Welfare of Cripples (later to become the International Society for Prosthetics and Orthotics), together with the International Association of Orthotists and Prosthetists (INTERBOR), have promoted the speedy exchange of information internationally. As a result surgeons and therapists are better informed and the modern prosthetist is not just craft-trained at the bench but technically trained, using techniques and devices from many countries.

It has taken time for the fruits of this programme to become general practice and the process of change still continues. Until 1960 most artificial limbs were 'exoskeletal': that is to say, they were hollow with an external frame shaped to resemble the body-shape through which the forces from the hand or foot were transferred to the body. Such a method of construction has its uses, but most prostheses are now 'endoskeletal', with a central post through which the force is transferred, shape being supplied by a purely cosmetic cover. Up to 1960 artificial limbs were mostly fabricated from wood, leather or aluminium – materials which still have their uses – and had changed little over the years. The prostheses for below-knee amputation were similar to those used in the Middle Ages or even Roman times. The above-knee prostheses closely resembled that supplied to the Marquis of Angelsey after the Battle of Waterloo, and was named after him. The prosthesis for hip disarticulation was little different from that described by Hoffe in 1891. Upper-limb prostheses resembled those described in the 1860s.

Since 1960 the results of the research programmes initiated in many countries have begun to come into use and progress has continued. Better understanding of prosthetic needs has led to improved amputation techniques, better engineering has led to better devices to replace human functions, better materials have resulted in improved fit, lightness, a more natural appearance, and the revival of good ideas which failed because of the unsuitable materials used in the past.

Until the problems of leaving artificial materials permanently transfixing the skin have been solved, the principles of amputation techniques and the transfer of forces across the interface between the body and the socket remain well established. The desirable functions of mechanisms to replace body functions are largely known but have yet to be fully achieved. Some mechanisms are too costly for all but a few patients, and other devices which are suitable for one culture are unacceptable for another. For instance, the knee flexion and ankle plantar flexion which is satisfactory to the Westerner is unacceptable to the follower of Islam, and the Japanese require a rotary element at the knee which Europeans do not need.

Particular mention must be made of electrically powered and controlled upper-limb prostheses which are now standard for selected patients in some countries. Development is progressing fast in all countries, but their use has largely developed because of the introduction of better and lighter power-packs and lighter, quieter, small electric motors from the space programme.

Examples of prostheses used to illustrate this book are largely taken from United Kingdom practices. Some have originated in the UK, but many are derived from principles originating elsewhere, although often modified. The reader should look for the underlying principles and choose those materials and components available which most nearly allow these criteria to be met.

The science and art of amputation and prosthetics have changed and are continuing to change. There is reason to believe that the future will see further advances leading to changes in amputation surgery, socket configuration, and controls. These possible advances are discussed in a later chapter.

In conclusion, the following is a short outline of some of the major changes in amputations and external limb prosthetics since the end of the Second World War.

Amputation, in which skill and speed used to be a matter of pride, had come to be regarded by many surgeons as a sign of failure and a last resort to be avoided if possible. Now most amputations are by surgeons who use amputation as the treatment of choice when it is indicated, representing a major change of attitude towards the procedure.

New materials and advances in prosthetic design have inspired the use of new surgical techniques or the revival of old ones. Disarticulation at the ankle, which had been modified surgically in the past to overcome prosthetic difficulties, is once again favoured because the appearance of the modern prostheses is acceptable to most patients except the young and fashion-conscious. The prostheses are of two main types. One is a plastic socket made to the contours of the stump, into which the stump is introduced from the back or the side; this originates from a concept developed by McLaurin of Canada. The other is tubular in shape with a foam or other compliant liner to the shape of the stump, through which the stump can be pushed. Both have their advantages but both are lighter, and of better apppearance, than the artificial limbs previously in use.

Disarticulation at the knee also was not favoured because a long anterior flap failed to heal and because the knee joint could not be replaced at knee-joint level within the contours of the natural limb, but had simple uniaxial joints on either side. Now the surgical problem has been overcome by the use of lateral flaps, and the prosthetic problem by the use of a four-bar linkage knee joint which can be placed below the knee to give a centrode of rotation at knee level.

The idea originated some time ago. Knee joints using four-bar linkage were devised by Stabilax in France, Polymatic in the USA, and the OFA in Sweden. All had disadvantages – weight, excessive stability, breakages etc. — which militated against their use. In 1969 one was developed in Denmark which gained some use and there is now one in general use in the UK which can accept the torques to which it is subjected.

Amputation through the shafts of long bone, which is the commonest amputation, has also changed since the Second World War. Whereas formerly muscles were allowed to retract, it is now considered that they should be reattached at normal muscle fibre length and tension to preserve as much of the residual power and vascular bed as possible.

In below-knee amputations, Hepp, Dederich and others in Germany, and Loon in the USA, favoured the osteomyoplastic amputation based on a technique used by Jackson Burrows after the First World War. The technique is still used but has largely been replaced by the long posterior flap. The latter was described by Verduyn in 1695 (Fig. 1.3) but had been long forgotten until revised by Kendrick in the UK in 1954. Burgess of Seattle further developed and popularized it in the 1960s and it is now the amputation most generally used worldwide at this level. It has been particularly successful in preserving useful below-knee amputation stumps in vascular disease. The most significant change at this level was the patellar-tendon-bearing prosthesis which Radcliffe and Foote developed at Berkeley and introduced in the early 1960s. This has given greatly improved load-bearing and has enabled patients to abandon thigh corsets and side steels. Its use has been spread throughout the world whether in its original form or with minor modifications particularly of the methods of suspension made in the USA, France, Germany, Denmark, UK and elsewhere.

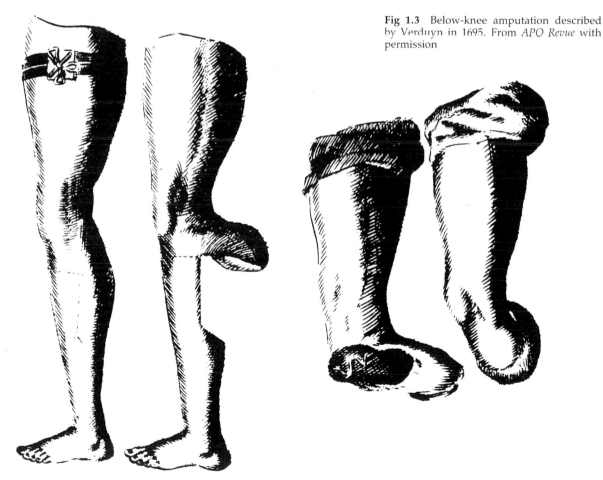

Fig 1.3 Below-knee amputation described by Verduyn in 1695. From *APO Revue* with permission

The myoplastic amputation has become the norm for mid-thigh amputation, a technique which has improved the vascularity and the power of the stump. It has also reduced the incidence of stump pain. This amputation is particularly suitable for new sockets. Whereas at the end of the Second World War the stump was introduced into an open-ended socket with a circumferential plug fit at the top, the modern sockets are closed at the bottom and in total contact with the stump while taking the axial load proximally on specific areas, in particular the ischial tuberosity. This has enabled pressure differential or 'suction' sockets to be widely used for active patients with a steady weight. There have also been advances in swing-and-stance phase controls which have greatly improved gait patterns. New materials have also helped to make these limbs lighter and to improve their appearance.

Disarticulation at the hip is relatively uncommon but is more frequent than it used to be. At the end of the Second World War, the patient sat in a socket fitting round the hemipelvis. This was perched over a hip joint vertically below the hip. This joint was locked to provide stability when standing, and when sitting was 7.5 cm (3 in) or more below the ischium, causing a pelvic tilt. McLaurin of Canada made a socket embracing the whole pelvis, thus dispensing with the shoulder harness, and placed the hip joint antero-inferiorly at the level of the normal joint, which is stable when standing and allows hip movement in the swing phase.

The principles of surgery in the upper limb are similar to those in the lower limb. There have been considerable advances in making artificial arms lighter and of better appearance. There have been minor improvements in the use of prostheses but there is much need for further development of mechanical usage as well as sensory feedback. The important improvements have been in socket fit, and in particular the socket brim suspension of the below-elbow prosthesis pioneered at Munster and modified at North Western University. These sockets have facilitated the use of electrical power and myoelectric controls. The use of electrical power with either mechanical or myoelectrical controls is now practised at many centres and is developing fast. Smidl in Italy uses it widely for adults, and other countries using electrical power in selected cases include Russia, Sweden, Yugoslavia, USA, Canada, Japan, as well as the UK. It is, however, as yet in its infancy.

The above is only a brief outline of the many advances being made throughout the world. The surgeon and the prosthetist are working in a field which can draw upon the past but is also advancing steadily into the future. This book tries to give the basic principles of surgery and prosthetic techniques which can be applied worldwide at the present time but which, with advances in materials and medicine, may need to change. These principles are illustrated largely from UK practice, but practitioners should apply them while using the materials and mechanisms available to them which most nearly meet the need.

2

Statistics and Trends

The number of people who undergo amputation and survive to have and to use a prosthesis of any kind depends upon the types of disease present in the population and the quality of medical care available. In primitive societies, with little or no medical care, the unfortunate either die or continue to drag out an existence carrying the burden of their disability. As these societies develop and medical aid becomes available the indigenous diseases are those most needing treatment. With the gradually increasing use of machinery for agriculture, industry, and transportation, there is a proportional increase in the incidence of trauma involving the arms and the legs, many such injuries leading to amputation. In the highly developed industrial nations the expectation of life is higher despite the increased complexities of life, and the number of traumatic amputations and degenerative diseases in which people outlive their limbs is becoming a major problem.

Statistics on the number and causes of amputations are not easily available from developing countries. Many of the estimates which have been published are based either on too few numbers or on unrepresentative samples. Even today it is not possible to give accurate figures for the number and causes of amputation in the population of any large nation. Most of the combatant nations in the two World Wars have produced well-documented figures about service and civilian casualties, but only in the past 20 years have they shown an interest in preparing similar information about their peacetime civilian population.

Since 1957 the health authorities in England and Wales have kept fairly detailed records of all new amputees referred to their Limb-Fitting Centres; this is probably the largest existing survey of a total population. The records do not, however, include the considerable number of amputees who have not been referred to the Limb-Fitting Centres, and are therefore to this extent incomplete. However, the statistics produced from England and Wales do correlate very closely in general terms with peacetime figures from European and American sources, giving useful information regarding the extent and depth of the problem.

In any study of statistics relative to amputations it is necessary to differentiate between amputation and amputee inasmuch as one amputee may have suffered the loss of more than one limb. Likewise it is not possible to correlate the number of amputations recorded in hospital operating-theatre books because these may record digital ablations in addition to reamputations on the same patient.

Unfortunately, in the world as a whole, war is still a major cause of limb loss; injury, both traffic and industrial, is common in populations recently exposed to modern technology. Disease, in particular tropical diseases and leprosy, is also a major cause in many parts of the world. As yet, therefore, statistics from developed countries cannot be applied to those countries that are not so well developed.

Amputation was formerly an infrequent operation in peacetime. Muirhead Little quotes EM Corner of St Thomas' Hospital, London, as reporting that in 1913 there were 5403 operations in that hospital of which only 34 were amputations. Little also states that the Royal Surgical Aid Society, a charitable organization for the needy, had only supplied 384 artificial legs compared with 39 290 other surgical appliances in 1915. He compared this with the 41 050 British service amputees from the First World War, 26 262 of whom were treated at Roehampton. The number of amputations among service casualties was much lower in the Second World War although civilian casualties were considerably higher, about 20 000 being treated at Roehampton. The type of warfare in which the British troops were involved probably accounts in part for this reduction in amputations, but improved techniques and the relearning of the advantages of delayed primary suture, the improved medical services and the advent of bacteriostatic and antibiotic preparations, undoubtedly all played their part.

The Limb-Fitting Services of England and Wales cooperate closely and provide prostheses almost without exception for all who are eligible under the National Health Service (NHS), including war pensioners and also servicemen who may lose a limb in the service of their country. In England and Wales close to 5000 new amputees are seen each year. The total number of patients referred to Limb-Fitting Centres for the first time each year from 1961 to 1984 is given in Fig. 2.1 and shows an increase of 66% built up over the intervening years.

The total number of amputees who were seen at centres in England and Wales in 1982, who were below the age of 60 years expressed as a percentage of the whole, was 24.9% compared with 49.1% in 1961. The ratio of arm amputations to leg amputa-

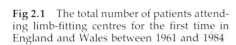

Fig 2.1 The total number of patients attending limb-fitting centres for the first time in England and Wales between 1961 and 1984

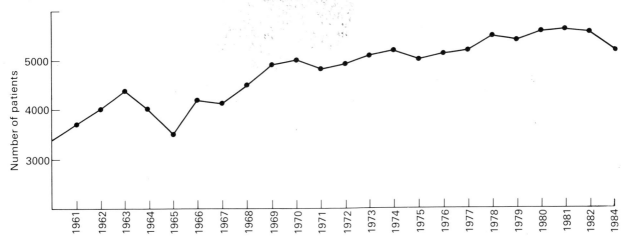

Table 2.1 Total number of patients seen in Limb-Fitting Centres for the first time in 1982

	Male	Female	Total*	
Single arm amputations	137	55	192	(201)
Double arm amputations	1	0	1	(3)
	138	55	193	(204)
Single leg amputations	3161	1649	4810	(4644)
Double leg amputations	133	54	187	(193)
Totals	3294	1703	4997	(4837)
Double arm amputations, previously single	0	0	0	(1)
Double leg amputations, previously single	248	75	323	(338)
Multiple amputations	8	3	11	(12)
Non-amputation patients (referred for advice/ prosthetic management)	104	79	183	(180)
Totals	3792	1915	5707	(5575)

*Figures in parentheses represent totals for 1981

tions changed from 1 : 11 in 1961 to 1 : 26 in 1982. The total number of patients seen for the first time in 1982 is shown in Table 2.1.

The change is accounted for by the steady increase in the numbers of elderly people suffering from the diseases of old age, especially atherosclerosis and diabetes. Amputations for peripheral vascular disease account for 62.5% of all cases referred to Limb-Fitting Centres. The other conditions that result in limb ablation are shown in Fig. 2.2.

The breakdown of vascular aetiology in patients referred during 1982 shows that arteriosclerosis was responsible for 86.1% of amputations, embolism for 7.4%, thromboangiitis for 1.1%, varicose ulceration for 2.4%, and other vascular conditions for 3%.

Road-traffic accidents accounted for nearly twice as many amputations (37%) as industrial injuries (19.4%). Of the 204 amputations performed in 1982 in consequence of road-traffic accidents, 165 involved the rider or the passenger of a powered two-wheel vehicle. Accidents in the home resulted in 47 amputations, or 8.5% of the total caused by trauma, while only 6.7% resulted from service with the Armed Forces.

In lower-limb amputations there is a welcome and increasing trend towards preserving the natural knee joint whenever possible, even in cases of diabetic gangrene and atherosclerosis. In 1961 the proportion of above-knee amputations to below-knee amputations (excluding those above the lesser trochanter and those distal to the ankle joint) at centres in England and Wales was 3 : 1; in 1981 it had fallen to 3 : 2 (in percentage terms 59% to 41%). However this figure is still well below the achievement of certain specialist centres, where the percentage of below-knee

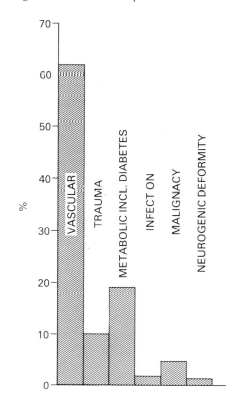

Fig 2.2 Reasons for amputation

amputations for peripheral vascular disease and diabetes mellitus is over 70%.

There is a disparity between the sexes, with the male-to-female ratio of 2.8 : 1 in 1961 decreasing to 3 : 1 in age groups below the age of 60 years, with a continuing tendency to parity in age groups over 60.

Of greater importance than the numbers referred to Limb-Fitting Centres are the numbers who are satisfactorily fitted with prostheses. In the lower-limb amputee, evaluation of success depends much on the observer. Since early history amputees have been rendered independent with crude surgery and simple prostheses that give no more than equalization of leg length, so that restoration of mobility to a young amputee is no criterion of surgical or prosthetic excellence. It is some indication of success, however, if the mobility of an older patient can be restored, or even improved. The relief from ischaemic pain and the restoration of body image can be a great boost to the morale of an elderly person, and a motivation to achieve a high degree of rehabilitation.

Success in fitting upper-limb prostheses depends largely upon the degree of motivation of the particular patient. Of two patients of similar age and disability who have achieved equal skill in using the arm prosthesis after training, only one will use it constantly; the other will reject it. The Liverpool Limb-Fitting Centre reported on the use made of their prostheses by upper-limb amputees attending that Centre (Table 2.2). Clearly arm

Table 2.2   The use of the split hook appliance by amputees (1973)

Amputation	Sex	No.	Split hook used		
			Regularly	Occasionally	Never
Elective					
Above-elbow	M	94	7 (7.5%)	22 (23.5%)	65 (69%)
	F	9	—	—	9 (100%)
Below-elbow	M	169	28 (16.4%)	42 (24.8%)	99 (58%)
	F	44	1 (2%)	2 (4.5%)	41 (93.5%)
All levels	M	263	35 (13%)	64 (24%)	164 (62%)
	F	53	1 (1.9%)	2 (3.7%)	50 (94%)
Both sexes	M/F	316	36 (11.3%)	66 (20.8%)	214 (67%)
Congenital	M	20	3 (15%)	5 (20.8%)	12 (60%)
	F	34	—	—	34 (100%)

prostheses are of general use for only a small number of patients, have a limited use (mainly cosmetic) for a much larger number, and are totally rejected by others.

It is interesting to note that of 211 myoelectric arms issued to children aged four years and over, beginning in 1978 and continuing up to the present, 82% are still in active use. It is expected that within the next five years myoelectric arms will become available for all below-elbow amputees and selected above-elbow amputees of all ages.

Table 2.3. Outcome of lower limb amputations in England, Wales and Northern Ireland, 1973*

Category	% fitted and satisfactory after training	% of all patients fitted
All	76.3	68.9
Single amputees	76.5	69.0
Bilateral amputees	72.3	68.2
Aged 60–79	73.3	68.2
Aged 80+	63.8	60.0

*Prostheses were fitted to 77.6% of all amputees; non-fitment was due to death, senility or intercurrent disease in the remainder.

Table 2.3 shows the outcome of lower-limb amputees and presents a somewhat better picture than Table 2.2. Results are considered satisfactory if patients in their seventies or eighties are able to move independently in their own homes. Inevitably at that age many die or succumb to intercurrent illness but these figures show that even for the very old there is considerable hope of success.

The analysis of the figures for new patients, which of course includes geriatric patients with a short life expectancy, is not indicative of the numbers and types of amputees who are in the community. In 1982 there were over 65 000 amputees in England and Wales which have a combined population of approximately 50 000 000: of these some 14 000 were war pensioners (over 2000 being from the First World War) and the remainder were civilians with both long standing and recent amputations

Table 2.4 Age distribution of patients seen for the first time in two successive years 1981 and 1982

Age (years)	1981	%	1982	%
0 – 9	33	0.61	36	0.65
10 – 19	178	3.30	160	2.90
20 – 39	268	4.97	338	6.12
40 – 59	970	17.99	824	14.92
60 – 79	3243	60.15	3411	61.74
over 80	700	12.98	755	13.67

In a limited survey of 600 patients (aged 18 or over) attending the Roehampton Limb-Fitting Centre, carried out by the Biomechanical Research and Development Unit in 1969 (Table 2.5), it was found that 32% of patients had suffered amputation before 1940 and a further 4% before 1910. The longevity of these earlier amputees, mostly from the First World War, is indicative that trauma was the prime cause of amputation within the first four decades of life.

From this it is clear that the amputee population of England and Wales comprises three broad categories of amputees.

1 Those who lose a limb in childhood, adolescence, or early

Table 2.5. Date of first amputation in 600 amputees over 18

Decade of amputation	Cases (%)	
1909 or before	4	
1910–19	10	32
1920–29	9	
1930–39	9	
1940–49	24	
1950–1959	15	68
1960–69	29	

adult life and whose life expectancy is long form the first category. These are the active amputees for whom the Limb Service will be responsible for many years; their numbers increase each year, and they require a different prosthetic approach and management from the other groups.

2 The second category comprises those who suffer amputation because of degenerative diseases that are more common in the sixth and subsequent decades of life, where life expectancy is reduced and whose total numbers over the years remain fairly constant. The number of such new patients each year corresponds closely to the natural wastage in the group.

3 The smallest group comprises patients who suffer amputation because of malignant disease or as a result of congenital or acquired limb malformation.

Artificial-limb construction and supply needs to be varied for each of the above groups. For the active amputee the prosthesis must be functional, durable, and of good appearance, and, above all, manufactured and fitted as soon as possible after amputation. For the elderly the weight of the prosthesis becomes the prime factor in ensuring success, but it must still be cosmetically acceptable. Where limb ablation has a poor prognosis, very early fitting and delivery must take priority over all other considerations.

Table 2.6 represents a survey of 1000 patients who were seen on a routine basis at one of the Roehampton Limb-Fitting Clinics in 1984; age groups and cause of amputation are detailed. (Patients seen on second or subsequent visits are excluded.)

It is evident that the major cause of amputation today is atherosclerosis, but the cause of limb loss in those who continue to attend Limb-Fitting Centres for many years is mainly injury. Congenital deformities of limbs leading to amputation or to the need for special extension prostheses constitute a numerically smaller group requiring treatment over many years.

Over the years it has become evident that an elderly person who loses a leg through atherosclerosis in the seventh or eighth decade of life, and who survives for three to seven years will probably also lose the remaining leg. For this reason alone every effort should be made by the surgeon to preserve the natural knee at the first amputation.

Table 2.6 Survey of 1000 patients seen at a Roehampton Limb-Fitting Clinic in 1984

| Age (years) | Cause of amputation | | | |
	Trauma	Vascular disease	Congenital	Other
0 – 9	2	0	16	14
10 – 19	32	2	14	
20 – 39	86	8	12	41
40 – 59	111	62	8	67
60 – 79	27	371	2	63
Over 80	3	31	0	5
Totals	261	474	52	213

3

Human Locomotion and Prosthetics

This chapter is intended to provide the reader with an understanding of the purposes and actions of prostheses; it deals only superficially with those in common use. The reader who wishes to know more on the subject is advised to consult the textbooks listed on pages 218–220.

A prosthesis has three major parts: (a) the interface consisting of the stump-socket complex, additional suspension, and body-operated controls; (b) the 'skeleton' which replaces the lost limb segments and is used as a system of connecting links between the artificial joints; and (c) the artificial joints which, in order to mimic the natural joints, have devices to limit, modify, or assist their movements.

All movement in a lower-limb prosthesis, and much of it in an upper-limb prosthesis, even in those with external power, is imparted by the stump via the stump-socket interface. The design of the stump is the responsibility of the surgeon, while the prosthetist is responsible for fashioning the socket.

The skeleton provides a system of levers by which power is transmitted to the joints of the living limb and by which they are largely controlled. The residual amputation stump normally is itself a lever that provides the power which acts through the stump-socket interface on the mechanisms. The length of these levers, their adjustment (particularly in the lower limb), and their weight distribution, as well as their total weight, need to be considered if the function of the prosthesis is to be understood.

THE LOWER LIMB

The leg is a jointed strut that supports the mass of the body weight in standing or walking. The various joints allow the necessary movements of the strut during the gait cycle.

The gait

The features of the patient's walk, or gait pattern, may be examined by clinical observation and by an analysis of the interactions of the forces and movements taking place at the major joints of the limb.

Clinical observation shows that the normal human gait has certain consistent features. With each stride there is a vertical rise and fall and a horizontal medial lateral sway of the body of about 5 cm (2 in) in each direction. There is some pelvic rotation about a vertical axis. The stride lengths are symmetrical and measure about 76–81 cm (30–32 in). The average number of steps per minute – the step cadence – is about 90–110. The above facts indicate that the average speed of walking is about 4 km/h (2.5 mph).

An examination of the interaction of forces and movements taking place at the major joints of the lower limb provides a more precise analysis of the gait cycle than can be achieved by simple clinical observation. One complete gait cycle is defined as the period between two successive heel strikes by the same foot. This period is divided into two parts. The first part is the stance phase. This starts with 'heel-strike' and ends when the toe of the same foot leaves the ground. The second part of the gait cycle is the swing phase. This starts with 'toe-off' (when the big toe leaves the ground) and ends when the heel of the same foot strikes the ground again. The swing and stance phases of the gait cycle may be subdivided as shown in Fig. 3.1.

During normal walking the swing phase of one leg coincides with the stance phase of the other leg. However there is some overlap during which both feet are on the ground. This period is known as the 'double-support time'. The double-support period of the gait cycle disappears when the subject starts to run. At ordinary walking speeds each leg is in stance phase for about 60% and in swing phase for about 40% of its gait cycle. The period of double support occupies about 25% of the average gait-cycle time and is made up of a portion of the stance-phase time for each leg.

The following account is taken from the paper on *Human Locomotion* presented by Edward Peizer and Donald W Wright at a symposium on *Prosthetic and Orthotic Practice* held in Dundee, Scotland, June 1969. (Reproduced with permission from E. Peizer and D.W. Wright (1970) Human Locomotion. In G. Murdoch (ed) *Prosthetic and Orthotic Practice*, pp. 24–36. London: Edward Arnold.)

Analysis of motions and forces

With this background we can turn our attention to the specific motions which occur at the joints to produce a characteristic gait and the forces which produce those motions. Motion at the joints of each segment of the body results from the interaction of two sets of forces: internal forces which are produced inside the body by the muscles, and external forces

Fig 3.1 Gait cycle. (a) Stance phase, (b) Swing phase. From E. Peizer and D.W. Wright (1970), with kind permission of the publisher, Edward Arnold

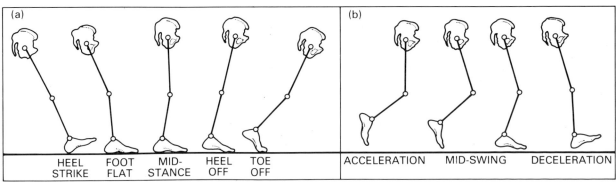

(a)					(b)		
HEEL STRIKE	FOOT FLAT	MID-STANCE	HEEL OFF	TOE OFF	ACCELERATION	MID-SWING	DECELERATION

represented principally by the influence of gravity on the body. We move about in a sea of gravity which is constantly trying to pull each segment of the body toward the ground. Muscles inside the body are generating forces which resist gravity and modulate it in a way that permits walking as well as other activities.

The force of gravity is not always antagonistic nor does it always act as an impediment or a resistance to be overcome. On the contrary, gravity aids us in initiating gait. In standing erect a vertical projection of the centre of gravity falls anterior to the hip joint tending to flex it, anterior to the knee joint tending to extend it, and anterior to the ankle joint tending to dorsiflex it. We therefore stand by the combined action of the plantar flexors of the ankle and the extensors of the hip. Normally, to begin walking we relax the plantar flexors of one leg allowing the body to fall forward on that side, and swing the other leg forward at the hip.

Let us now consider the forces and motions at each of the major joints during walking. The significant events are best reviewed in three planes.

Sagittal plane

The significant activity taking place at the ankle, knee and hip joints in the sagittal plane is shown in Figs 3.2, 3.3. and 3.6. In the upper portion of Fig. 3.2. is a representation of the lower limb and the relationships among the three major joints as each of five key gait events occur – heel contact, foot flat, mid-stance, heel-off and toe-off. The next section down shows the changed position of the ankle joint as it rotates immediately after heel contact. The forces tending to rotate the ankle are represented along the same time base in the section labelled 'ankle moment'.

These data indicate a highly transient, low order dorsiflexion moment about the ankle, immediately after heel contact, representing the 'dig' of the heel as it strikes the ground. As increasing amounts of body weight are transmitted to the ground, reaction forces pushing back up against the heel create a moment tending to plantar flex the ankle. Just before the sole of the shoe touches the ground (foot flat) the peak plantar flexion moment is reached at approximately 10% of the cycle. This is followed very rapidly by the peak plantar flexion angle of the ankle of approximately 15–20° which occurs under the influence of the peak ankle moment of 24 to 27 Nm (newton metre) (18 to 20 ft lb). The ground reaction force causes motion about the ankle at a rate governed by the dorsiflexors of the ankle (principally tibialis anticus) which absorb the force of the moment by stretching, and allows the ankle to move into plantar flexion.

With the foot flat, and for the present immovable, the mass of the body above the ankle joint rotates about it, changing the direction of ankle motion from plantar flexion to dorsiflexion. As both the swinging leg and a vertical projection of the body's centre of gravity move anteriorly, a large moment is generated about the ankle joint tending to move it in the direction of dorsiflexion. The peak dorsiflexion moment is reached very shortly after heel-off, when the vertical projection of the centre of gravity is well out in front of the ankle joint and the full body weight is being carried on the stance foot. In normal walking, moments between 81 and 108 Nm (60 and 80 ft lb), tending to drive the ankle into dorsiflexion, have been recorded. Under these moments the ankle moves from a position of maximum plantar flexion to a position of maximum dorsiflexion of approximately 15° just before the heel-off. The rate at which the ankle rotates to maximum dorsiflexion is governed by the gastrocnemius, whose eccentric contraction controls the motion of the ankle into

Fig 3.2   Ankle kinetics (1.3558 ft lb = 1 Nm).
From E. Peizer and D.W. Wright (1970), with
kind permission of the publisher, Edward
Arnold

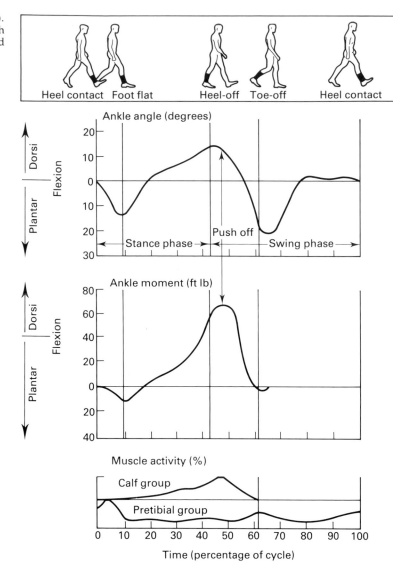

dorsiflexion and limits it just before heel-off. Forcible contraction of the
gastrocnemius rapidly reverses the direction of the ankle motion from a
position of maximum dorsiflexion to a position approximating maximum
plantar flexion at toe-off. This is accompanied by a rapidly diminishing
dorsiflexion moment about the ankle.

At the instant of toe-off the ankle is in approximately 15° of plantar
flexion. During the swing phase of gait it returns to approximately 90°
where it is found at the instant of the next heel contact. Thus the ankle
rotates through a total excursion of approximately 90° during each stance
and swing phase.

The controlling influence of the anterior and posterior leg muscles is,
of course, lost in amputation. Single-axis prosthetic feet are usually
equipped with both plantar flexion and dorsiflexion bumpers whose

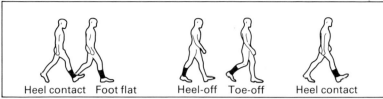

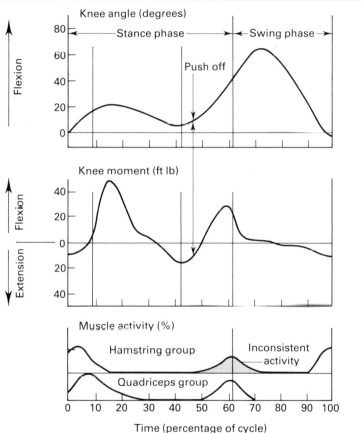

Fig 3.3   Knee kinetics (1.3558 ft lb = 1 Nm). From E. Peizer and D.W. Wright (1970), with kind permission of the publisher, Edward Arnold

resilience absorbs the moments tending to rotate the ankle. Their function is only partly analogous to the muscles. Resilient bumpers or springs have a reasonably constant load versus deflection curve and do not respond adequately to moments generated in walking. They require patients to adapt their gaits to the properties of the bumpers in order to obtain a semblance of the normal motion about the ankle joint. In case of paralysis of the muscles controlling the ankle, we are all familiar with 'drop foot' as a result of weakened tibialis muscles which become incapable of absorbing moments tending to plantar flex the ankle and permit it to go from heel contact to foot flat too rapidly with audible effects.

As shown in Fig. 3.3, the motions and the forces acting about the knee also demonstrate a characteristic pattern. Immediately after heel contact we note a transient, low magnitude extension moment about the knee

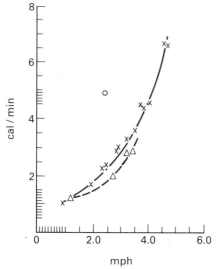

Fig 3.4   Net energy costs of several locomotion modes. (Key: X ——, normal subjects; O, above-knee amputee; △ – – –, wheelchair propulsion.) (1 mile = 1.61 km) from E. Peizer and D.W. Wright (1970), with kind permission of the publisher, Edward Arnold

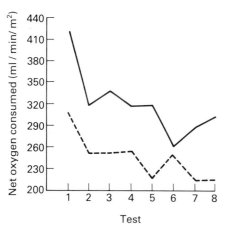

Fig 3.5   Energy cost of restricted knee movement recorded under a number of test conditions (1–8) representing various levels of exercise. From E. Peizer and D.W. Wright (1970), with kind permission of the publisher, Edward Arnold

which represents the 'dig' or backward movement of the leg; after overshooting the ground at the extreme end of the swing phase, it falls back into contact with the ground. Immediately thereafter, with the heel in contact with the ground and increasing amounts of body weight being applied through the leg, the ground reaction line passes behind the knee centre, creating a substantial moment of approximately 68 Nm (50 ft lb) at the time of foot flat. The activity of the quadriceps muscles resists the moment, and by stretching permits the knee to flex to approximately 20° in early stance. The flexion moment diminishes rapidly after foot flat, as the mass of the body above the ankle rotates forward, reducing the distance between the centre of the knee rotation and the line of the ground reaction force. The instant of mid-stance is indicated by the zero moment about the knee occurring at approximately 32% of the stance phase after which an extension moment is generated, with a peak of approximately 20 Nm (15 ft lb) as the knee becomes fully extended again just prior to heel-off. At the time of heel-off the knee begins to flex again and as its centre of rotation moves further anterior to the ground reaction line, the flexion moment about the knee reaches a secondary peak of approximately 27 Nm (20 ft lb) and returns to zero at the instant of toe-off.

The pattern of gait is radically altered in the absence of the knee due to amputation. The absence of the musculature controlling the knee severely reduces the ability to absorb the normal knee moments. The above-knee amputee compensates by shortening his step to prevent the development of a large moment tending to flex the knee, or by leaning forward at the hip and preventing the ground reaction line from passing behind the knee, in order to reduce or reverse the direction of the moment generated. Nevertheless, when his heel strikes the ground, a moment tending to flex the knee is generated and the amputee resists it by extension of the hip. In addition to the observable anomalies of the gait that these manoeuvres cause, perhaps the most significant result is that normal knee flexion in early stance is impossible. The knee remains fully extended over perhaps 45% of the stance phase. This means that the vertical oscillation of the centre of gravity will have a greater-than-normal magnitude, increasing the work done in walking and the energy required. Previous studies have shown that above-knee amputees require approximately 100% more energy to walk than normal people (Fishman et al., 1962) (Fig. 3.4). A significant portion of this excess is doubtlessly due to the inability to flex the knee in early stance. The same study showed that in a highly trained, normal individual the restriction of normal knee movement in early stance increased energy consumption by approximately 25% (Fig. 3.5).

During the swing phase of gait, forcible hip flexion accelerates the knee centre. Due to their inertia, the leg and foot tend to lag behind the accelerating knee centre, producing flexion about the knee which reaches approximately 65° and then begins to extend, reaching full extension at the time of the next heel contact.

The characteristic pattern of normal hip motion is shown in Fig. 3.6. With the leg advanced at the instant of heel contact, the pelvis and the superincumbent mass remain approximately vertical, causing the hip to flex approximately 25°. In this position, as body weight is applied, the ground reaction force creates a flexion moment about the hip since its line of action passes behind the knee and ankle joints and just anterior to the hip joint. Just before foot flat a peak flexion moment of approximately 81 Nm (60 ft lb) is typical. As the major mass of the body rotates over the ankle and knee joints between foot flat and mid-stance, the ground

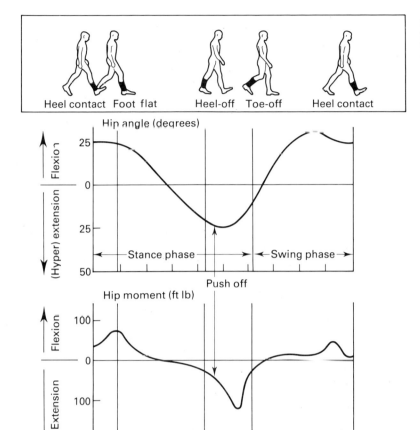

Fig 3.6   Hip kinetics (1.3558 ft 1b = 1 Nm). From E. Peizer and D.W. Wright (1970), with kind permission of the publisher, Edward Arnold

reaction force passes through and then behind the hip joint; the hip moment is zero when the reaction line passes through the joint. An extension moment about the hip is generated shortly after foot flat and gradually increases to approximately 54 Nn (40 ft lb) just before heel-off. The position of the hip has changed from approximately 25° of flexion at the beginning of stance phase to approximately 15° of extension (or hyperextension). Maximum extension of the hip is achieved just after heel-off when it reaches approximately 20°. Very shortly after this peak between heel-off and toe-off, and coinciding with the time of push-off, the peak extension moment about the hip is reached. Its magnitude is normally well over 136 Nm (100 ft lb). Shown in the bottom section of Fig. 3.6 is the related muscle activity. The peak activity of gluteus maximus and erector spinae muscles are seen to occur when the flexion moment about the hip is maximum. Their function at this time is to resist the flexion moment and prevent the torso from collapsing over the hip. Similar activity of both muscles, though of lesser magnitude, occurs just after heel-off and before push-off. Forcible plantar flexion is accompanied by a peak extension moment and maximum electrical activity of the gluteus maximus. The low peak of activity shown for the erector spinae at this time is probably due to their action in stabilizing the torso on the pelvis during the push-off.

Frontal plane

Viewed in the frontal plane, angular rotations of far less magnitude are seen than those in the sagittal plane. In discussing the clinically desirable factors of gait we have already pointed out that the hip rotates in the frontal plane and 'dips' approximately 4 or 5°. Maximum rotation occurs at approximately 12 to 15% of the stance phase or just before foot flat, when the maximum vertical load is being applied. Under rapid loading, the pelvis on the swing side tends to drop when its supporting member leaves the ground to initiate swing. At this instant, substantial moments are generated tending to adduct the hip joint. The magnitude of these moments has never been precisely measured; however, reasonable estimates made from photographic data indicate these moments to be of

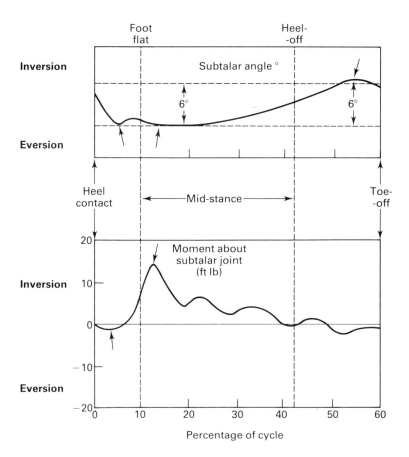

Fig 3.7 Subtalar kinetics (1.3558 ft lb = 1 Nm). From E. Peizer and D.W. Wright (1970), with kind permission of the publisher, Edward Arnold

the order of approximately 68 Nm (50 ft lb). The dip of the pelvis on the swing side is limited to 4 or 5° by the action of the abductors of the hip on the stance side. Once the rotation of the hip in the frontal plane has been limited and the period of mid stance occurs, the adduction moment about the hip drops very sharply. It begins to rise again from this point, rapidly approaching a peak of approximately 81 Nm (60 ft lb) at the time of push-off.

A similar pattern of bimodal peak moments occurs in the frontal plane about the knee. Since moments in the frontal plane are products of the ground reaction force, whose line of action passes from a point under the foot through the centre of gravity, all moments in the frontal plane will always be in the direction of adduction at hip and knee, and at the ankle principally in the direction of inversion. Although moments of approximately 27 to 41 Nm (20 to 30 ft 1b) tending to adduct the knee have been calculated, no rotation about the knee occurs in the frontal plane.

As shown in Fig. 3.7 the subtalar joint everts approximately 6° between heel contact and foot flat. It should be borne in mind that this is not to say that the *position* of the subtalar joint is in eversion. At the instant of heel contact the angle at the subtalar joint maintains the foot in a position of inversion. Immediately after heel contact the ground reaction force passes lateral to the subtalar joint and the foot is rotated from its initial position of inversion of approximately a neutral position, moving in the *direction* of eversion. This motion of the subtalar joint is accompanied by very low moments about the subtalar joint and initially is resisted principally by gravity. However, having rotated approximately 6°, and with a substantial amount of body weight applied at foot flat, a substantial moment of approximately 20 Nm (15 ft lb), tending to invert the foot, is generated. The foot is maintained in its approximately neutral position by the activity of the invertors. Although the inversion moment about the subtalar joint diminishes steadily until toe-off, the subtalar joint begins to invert in mid-stance, reaching a peak of approximately 6° just before toe-off. The precise kinematics of the subtalar joint in swing phase are not known, but the position of the subtalar joint is relatively inverted at the onset of each stance phase.

Transverse plane

A set of complex transverse rotations is known to take place in the pelvis, hip joint, femur and the tibia. The interrelationships among these rotations in the transverse plane have not been clarified. For the purpose of study, the net rotation of the lower extremity in the transverse plane is summed in the rotation of the tibia, for which reasonably adequate data are available. As shown in Fig. 3.8, from a 'neutral' position, that is, in a position of external or clockwise rotation at the instant of heel contact, the tibia rotates internally or counterclockwise rather rapidly. Very shortly after foot flat it reaches a peak of internal rotation of approximately 9° and begins to rotate slowly in the opposite or clockwise direction. Its rate of derotation, that is, in the clockwise direction, is approximately half the rate of internal rotation and the tibia returns to its neutral or starting point just after heel-off. The initial internal rotation of the tibia is accompanied by a very low moment of approximately 3 Nm (2 ft lb), since very little body weight has been applied up to that time. During the period of mid-stance (approximately 15 to 30% of the stance-phase time) the counterclockwise moment tending to rotate the tibia internally increases substantially *while the tibia actually rotates externally*. It is an apparent paradox for the tibia to move in the direction of external rotation while

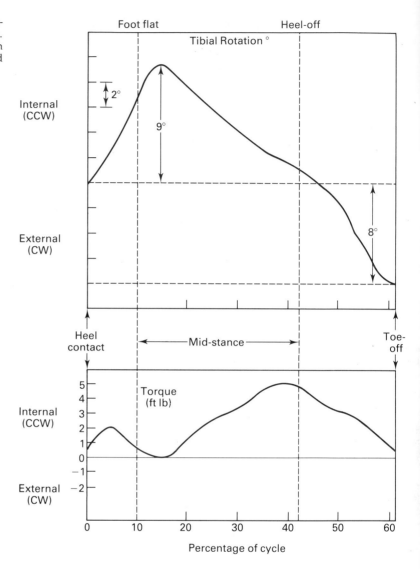

Fig 3.8 Tibial kinetics (CCW, counterclockwise: CW, clockwise) (1.3558 ft 1b = 1 Nm). From E. Peizer and D.W. Wright (1970), with kind permission of the publisher, Edward Arnold

the moment tending to rotate it internally increases. It is attributed to the composite effects of the motion of the pelvis, particularly the advance of the pelvis on the swing side, causing external rotation of the hip joint tending to increase the internal rotation moment. In effect, the internal hip rotators acting eccentrically, control the rate at which the hip externally rotates. At the same time, the centre of pressure under the foot has shifted to the ball, but still on the lateral side, tending to increase the internal rotation moment.

In the below-knee or above-knee amputee these kinetic factors of hip motion are still present. When the amputee walks in a prosthesis these forces are transmitted down through the prosthesis to the ground, tending to rotate it in the transverse plane, much as the normal tibia rotates. These rotations may be absorbed at the stump-socket interface where they create unwanted shear forces on tissue. They may cause shear or rotation between the foot and ground where they create instability. Compensatory manoeuvres frequently mask this primary cause since the patient will react by vaulting or circumduction, reducing the time he spends on the prosthetic leg, and by similar mechanisms which seem to indicate that the socket is uncomfortable. Without a careful analysis unnecessary adjustments of the socket may be made while the real remedy may lie elsewhere.

Energy considerations

All human activities are accomplished at a metabolic cost whose energy requirement is traditionally measured in units of oxygen consumed. By measuring oxygen consumption during an activity and comparing it to oxygen consumption during a similar period of rest, 'the net cost' of an activity can be determined. One of the most remarkable aspects of normal human locomotions is the extreme economy with which it is performed. The net energy cost of walking at normal speeds of approximately 4 km/h (2.5 mph) is roughly 10.5 J/min (2.5 cal/min) of walking. This is a net cost above that of simply sitting which is usually given at approximately 5 J/min (1.2 cal/min). In general, walking at speeds up to 6.5 km/h (4 mph) costs approximately 2.5 J/min per km/h (1 cal/min per mph). There is almost no other useful activity, e.g. typing, sweeping, dishwashing, playing a musical instrument, which can be accomplished at a significantly lower net energy cost. Common activities usually cost more, as for example, ironing clothes [12.5 J/min (3.0 cal/min)] and mopping floors [15 J/min (3.6 cal/min)].

Equally remarkable is the fact that in walking at speeds significantly below or above 'average' velocity, energy costs are significantly higher, a phenomenon which tends to support the theory that walking conforms to the minimum principle with respect to energy consumption. Normal gait is extremely efficient and any inefficiency, that is any alteration in the normal pattern of gait, decreases efficiency and increases energy consumption. A certain amount of support for this concept is seen in Fig. 3.4 in which are compared the energy costs for locomotion among normal subjects, above-knee amputees, and wheelchair users. Above-knee amputees require approximately twice the energy to walk at the same speeds as normal subjects. Wheelchair propulsion requires somewhat less energy than normal locomotion since two of the major energy-consuming factors of normal gait, vertical and horizontal oscillation of the centre of gravity, are eliminated.

Understanding locomotion as an energy-transforming process is a valuable tool in interpreting the needs of patients with impaired gait in relation to the mechanical systems which are provided them to restore more normal function. We have all observed the patient who walks quite normally in the clinic during his check-up and reverts to a lurching, limping, shambling gait outside the clinic when he is not 'on parade'. Is he lazy? Is he unaware of the poor appearance of his gait? Or, is it that in the clinic he demonstrated that he could walk in a reasonably normal manner in spite of his prosthesis? Did his reversion to a less normal appearing gait really mean that the energy required to walk normally in that prosthesis is too high to be maintained? This is a grim note upon which to conclude, but one that rings out the importance of a comprehensive understanding of locomotion for both clinicians and developers.

4

Principles of Prosthetic Design

The design of a limb prosthesis, whose purpose is to replace a missing limb and to restore or provide function, is largely governed by the level of amputation and the remaining function, although residual pathology or unrelated disease may also affect it. The patient's age, physique, balance, sight, environmental and psychological needs may be of far greater importance than the cause of amputation.

The natural functions that the prosthesis needs to restore are sensory input, voluntary motor action and psychological loss. Sensation is necessary to initiate, maintain and curtail voluntary motor action, whether it be an alarm-bell to wake us or the feel of an object we grasp. The psychological loss is usually referred to as body image, which is the shape, movement and consistency which each individual believes he has. This is not the only psychological loss, for involuntary movements such as clapping, stamping, etc., are emotional outlets which may also be lost through amputation.

A prosthesis should aim to replace in every respect the performance of the natural limb. The primary consideration for the user is a natural appearance in shape, texture and colour — motor function being of secondary importance. This desire for a natural appearance inhibits the use of designs which might provide prostheses with better engineering solutions to motor problems, such as tracked vehicles or telescopic arms. Prosthetic limb segments and joints must correspond to the equivalent natural levels.

The prime function of the lower limb is standing and walking. Other motor activities such as climbing, running, dancing, etc., are secondary. The lower limb is rarely used for sensory exploration of the environment, and the loss of epicritic sensation is therefore a minor disability. Also the lower limb is rarely used to express emotion.

In Westernized societies the lower limbs are normally covered by clothing and, providing the levels of joints and the general outline is a reasonable match, most patients do not need a faithful copy of the other limb.

For the upper limb the problem is much more complex: firstly because the motor function is much more varied in the power used and the movements of joints; secondly because the hand is important as a sense organ, exploring the environment by touch; and lastly because it is an important part of the body image. The hand is used in gesture as a supplement to speech, as an emotional outlet, and in personal contact, as well as being an important instrument in the intimacies of sexual relations.

Not only are the problems of restoring the loss of function less in the lower limb, but also the benefits conferred by a prosthesis are greater. When more than the foot and ankle are lost, locomotion is not possible without a mechanical aid, other than by hopping, but a device as crude as a crutch at once restores a high degree of mobility.

By contrast, one can lose the whole of an upper limb and still be able to wash, toilet, cook and eat, and follow many gainful and skilled occupations without any prosthesis. However, the gain from a prosthesis in body image, sensory feedback, and emotional outlet is poor, motor function is limited and crude, and to gain in appearance with a life-like hand is usually to forfeit some motor function.

There are many prosthetic devices that are useful but which do not resemble the human shape. There is still much to be done in prosthetic design, particularly of the upper limb, before such devices can be phased out and replaced by prostheses which are equally useful but also resemble human limbs.

For classification, prosthetic components fall into five major groups, namely:

1 interface components
2 terminal devices
3 joints, joint mechanisms and structure
4 cosmetic components
5 alignment devices

INTERFACE COMPONENTS

These are those parts of a prosthesis which are in direct contact with body tissues. Although a future development may be skeletal attachments and various control devices which penetrate the skin on a permanent basis, this type of prosthesis is not yet practical, and all contact between the prosthesis and the body is through the skin, which is therefore the body's interface component.

The prosthetic interface component is the socket for the stump, and any other component used to attach the prosthesis for suspension and voluntary control or to spread the workload. All the forces between the prosthesis and the body are transmitted through this interface.

The skin has a limited tolerance to pressure for both pain levels and vascularity, so the high forces which may be generated must be distributed over a wide area of skin, thus limiting even further the surface available for heat loss and direct contact with the environment. In multiple amputations the difficulty in losing heat can be considerable for someone living in a hot and humid climate and, because most materials currently used for sockets are impermeable, minimal enclosure of skin is desirable. Although the interface components prevent direct contact of the skin with the environment, some sensory information can be gathered by vibration and variation in the magnitude and direction of forces transmitted across the interface.

Ideally, all the functions of the interface to transmit the forces arising from the workload, attachment, and control of the prosthesis are contained in the socket. This ideal is achieved more often in modern prostheses, but ancillary load-bearing, suspension, and control harnesses are still necessary for many.

Socket

Definition. The socket has been defined as that part of the prosthesis into which the amputation stump is inserted, and the amputation stump as that part of the limb remaining below the most distal joint. Sockets may be made from any suitable available material. They may be carved from wood, moulded from leather, or shaped from metal. Today most sockets are made from plastic materials to a cast. Tissues deform under load and change form with movement. A simple wrap-cast of the stump does not therefore make a satisfactory socket unless the cast is modified by a skilled and experienced prosthetist. Methods of casting under static load have been devised for many levels which give better casts, but even these usually need adjustment — called rectification — by the prosthetist to give a satisfactory fit. This fit must be a comfortable compromise to all the shapes assumed by the stump in active use. A perfect fit in any one position is almost certainly a poor fit in other positions. A socket must be rigid or semi-rigid in those areas subjected to high loads, and most sockets have been uniformly made of the same material. Progress has been made in developing sockets with compliant areas which accept the changes under active use while retaining rigidity where it is needed.

Whatever the level of amputation, the socket gives circumferential pressure on the stump. These circumferential pressures are greater and more constant in the lower limb and in amputation through the shaft of long bones in which the major workload is proximal. They are much less than arterial pressure, but may be high enough to give significant impairment to venous and lymphatic return. Over a long period this impairment may lead to terminal congestion, peau d'orange, and eventually to an eczema-like condition of the unsupported soft tissues. It is most often seen in open-ended sockets or in those in which there is a chamber below the stump, particularly in the lower limb where gravity and hydrostatic pressure play their part. That it is not seen more often is in part due to compression of the air in a chamber below the stump by its piston-like action, even if the air eventually escapes, and in part to the support provided by a stump sock, worn by most amputees. It is now a widely accepted principle that whatever the site of the major loading on the stump there should be total contact with the socket, even if this contact be compliant. Total contact also gives better sensory input on spatial relations.

An intimate fit is desirable at all levels to give control of transverse forces which arise in the active use of both upper and lower limbs. These transverse forces cause high pressures at the upper and lower ends of the socket which become more highly concentrated if the socket is lax.

Lastly, there is the brim of the socket to consider. If there is an abrupt change from the forces at the interface and no forces acting on the skin, the soft tissue will lap over the brim and cause problems due to friction and impact. The brim of the socket should therefore be rounded or bevelled to give a gradual reduction and cessation of pressure.

Attachment of the prosthesis to the body, called suspension, is a function ideally performed by the socket. There are two ways of achieving this suspension: first by using pressure differential and second by using body contour.

The sockets using pressure differential are usually referred to as 'suction sockets', for the original concept was to maintain adhesion of the socket to the stump by providing an enclosed chamber below the stump in which an exhaust valve maintained at all times a pressure lower than atmospheric pressure. This 'negative' pressure, however, leads to congestion of the stump ends. It is now recognized that only such 'negative' pressure is necessary as will prevent distraction of the stump from the socket in the 'swing' phase, and that for much of the time it may be at or above atmospheric pressure.

Pressure differential is not possible as a means of suspension for the majority of patients, and suspension is then by body contour, which makes use of the shaping of the long bones at the ankle, knee, wrist or elbow, or the shapely waist or shoulder.

Pressure differential suspension is dependent upon the relation of stump and socket. Body contour suspension may be effected solely by the shape of the socket but often relies upon an auxiliary harness. Body contour suspension by the socket is most common in amputation by disarticulation at joints when the bulbous-ended stump is inserted into a socket shaped to the contours of the stump. This may be achieved by laying the stump into the socket through a lateral opening or by pushing it through a compliant inner liner shaped to the bulbous stump which is thrust into the socket from above.

Modern myoplastic stumps may achieve socket retention by muscular contraction. Sockets designed to make use of muscle action for suspension are called 'muscle-grab' sockets.

Amputation through the shafts of long bones does not provide a bony expansion producing a bulbous stump from which to suspend the prosthesis by the socket, and a bulbous stump without a bony substance is an embarrassment. The prosthesis must then be suspended from the bony expansion of the distal end of the long bone next above (or even from a higher level) by means of an extension of the socket. It is, however, still necessary to use supplementary harnessing at this level, or at a higher level if appropriate.

Controls

A prosthesis is controlled by the body through the interface, and for the best control there should be the closest fit, otherwise movement is lost. There are two types of control: one intrinsic, the other voluntary.

Intrinsic controls are operated by the musculature of the stump and the reactions of the prosthesis to the workload. These may be simple devices such as straps, elastic rebound, simple friction brakes, etc., or complex servo-mechanisms of the kind used in electrical hands to prevent slipping, but without too firm a grip. These mechanisms act automatically in response to the use of the prosthesis.

Voluntary controls are those which are operated at the will of the user. Some may also be simple, such as positioning the prosthesis in space using an optional locking device, or a simple cord from the shoulder to operate a hand device. They may also be very complex, such as the use of electrical impulses generated by muscles to control electrical devices. When practicable, these controls are sited within the socket; alternatively they may be sited outside the socket and held in place by suitable attachments.

Auxiliary load bearing

In some patients the stump is unable to sustain the full workload either because of the poor qualities of the stump tissues, the joint next above, or the musculature controlling that joint, or because of unusually high loads generated in a particularly high active use. In the lower limb this usually means transferring some of the load proximally to the area used in the next higher level of amputation. In the upper limb it may be necessary to prevent distraction of the prosthesis or to assist in maintaining a flexed position.

To summarize, there is an interface between the body and the prosthesis. Except for a minor, but important, use of sight and sound, the skin is the body's main interface component, and the prosthesis' interface is the socket, and any auxiliary suspensory or control harness. Control of the prosthesis depends on sensory perception, largely through the skin, and this is one reason why anaesthetic skin is a disadvantage. The forces generated in using the prosthesis are also transmitted through the interface. There are limits to the forces which healthy skin can tolerate, and scarred or anaesthetic skin are particularly vulnerable. The surgical procedure must first meet the pathological needs but, once this is satisfied, an understanding of the prosthetic needs in fashioning an amputation stump can improve the comfort of the amputee and the use of the prosthesis.

A prosthesis should cover as little of the body as possible so as not to be an encumbrance. The prosthetic interface must be large enough to distribute the load, making use of the area designed for impact, so that the forces across the interface can be tolerated, which involves not only providing an adequate area, but also directing the reaction. It must also provide as much sensory input as possible.

TERMINAL DEVICES

It can be argued that the terminal devices are part of the structure and mechanisms of the prosthesis and may include joints. They are the prosthetic representation of the hand and foot, which are the particular functioning parts of the limbs, and are therefore considered separately. Some are designed to resemble in appearance the natural hand or foot, with varying degrees of accuracy of shape, texture, and movement. These are described by the rather clumsy term 'anthropomorphic'. Others are designed solely for their functional use and bear no resemblance to the human hand or foot. These are termed 'non-anthropomorphic'. They can be very simple but effective devices, such as peg-legs and simple hooks, or highly complex, sophisticated devices, such as modern myoelectrically controlled powered hands.

Those cultures in which the foot is normally enclosed in a boot or shoe can use a variety of simple-shaped prosthetic feet which need a trained eye to detect in normal use. There are, however, many cultures in which open-toed shoes or sandals are worn, and a more realistic prosthesis is required (e.g. European women), not only for appearance but also for the actual attachment of certain types of sandal.

The prosthetic hand is a problem in all cultures. The hand has six types of prehension as well as being used to hold down or push. No mechanical device has yet been invented which can reproduce all these functions. The skin of the hand also changes colour, not only by exposure to sunlight but also in response to elevation or dependency. While gloves to cover a hand can be made to match the normal hand, the variations in skin tone of the normal hand cannot be duplicated. In practice it is common to provide a hand with limited function for appearance, but a split hook or other working tool for the active working usage.

Both foot and hand prostheses are discussed in greater detail in the appropriate chapters on upper and lower-limb prosthetics.

There is one further aspect of foot and hand prosthetics which needs consideration: namely, when the amputation is through the foot or hand. The standard prosthetic device cannot then be used and the socket must be included in the device itself.

The foot is not normally prehensile and its sensory importance is minor. A prosthetic device enclosing the foot has to withstand high forces in use which the materials currently available cannot withstand. There are advantages in retaining a sensory sole of the foot, etc., in some conditions, particularly in the elderly but the surgeon should consider the pros and cons carefully before embarking on a partial foot operation in an active patient for which a prosthesis giving a normal appearance cannot be provided. In contrast, unnatural as partial hand prostheses are in appearance, any sensory area of skin is of importance in the upper limb, and if there is this is an added bonus. With few exceptions, provided there is no anaesthesia, as much of the hand should be retained as possible, for it will be a better limb than any currently available prosthesis for a higher level.

JOINTS, JOINT MECHANISMS AND STRUCTURE

Structure

The structure of the prosthesis is that part which represents the segments of the natural limb between the joints, the terminal device, and the socket. There are two principal types of structure: 'exoskeletal' and 'endoskeletal'. These terms are used in relation to the structure of external limb prostheses, which are themselves 'exoprostheses'. There has been some confusion with implanted prostheses such as hip and knee replacements, which are 'endoprostheses'. The terms 'exo-' and 'endo-' are used in the present context in relation to the structure of the prosthesis. Until the past decade most artificial limbs were hollowed between the joints, the loads being transmitted directly by the materials, whether wood, leather, metal or plastic, giving the shape. This is now referred to as an 'exoskeletal' structure. Now many prostheses are made in which the workload is transmitted through a central post surrounded by a soft structure, which is solely concerned with appearance. This is referred to as 'endoskeletal'.

It is also appropriate at this point to clarify the term 'modular', which is much used and abused in the description of prostheses. A module is a standard measurement by definition. Sundry technical professions such as architecture have given the term a special technical meaning. Computer technology uses the term 'module' for a unit which is interchangeable. No prosthesis is fully 'modular' for even if the components of the prosthetic element of the interface are fabricated from standard parts, these have to be adjusted to fit each individual amputee. Most prostheses in modern times have had some components which are 'modular', in that a manufacturer would have within his own range components such as joints which could be exchanged in repair or maintenance.

The concept of 'modularity' of components has grown apace in the past 20 years, particularly with the modern use of 'endoskeletal exoprostheses'. There is now international as well as national agreement on the dimensions of many components, which allows for rapid maintenance in emergencies, and also of the use of items from different manufacturers at various levels. This is easier in the endoskeletal prostheses where there is international agreement on tube sizes, but is also possible for a limited number of the components of the exoskeletal prostheses.

There are advantages and disadvantages in the use of both

types of structure and in practice many prostheses are hybrid. In all prostheses where the workload is transmitted at the proximal part of the socket, the forces must be transmitted either through the material of the socket itself, which then functions as a structural element, or through an exoskeletal structure to support the socket. There must also be a minimal distance between the distal end of the socket, the next joint, and its mechanism below for an endoskeletal tube and its method of fixing to be used. The exoskeletal structure also provides a space, particularly in the upper limb, for housing power and control components within the dimensions of the limb. It could also be claimed, until the recent introduction of carbon fibre, that exoskeletal limbs were lighter than their endoskeletal counterparts. It is appropriate to point out here that, particularly in the lower limb, lightness is not always the prime consideration. In the upper limb the workload usually has an element of lifting against gravity to which is added the lifting of the prosthesis, so that lightness is of great importance, but the lower limb is swung in the same way as tennis rackets, golf clubs, cricket and base-ball bats, etc., in which weight distribution is an important factor. An ultra-light limb may also be difficult to control in windy conditions.

The endoskeletal structure gives greater flexibility in the adjustment of axial rotation of one segment of the prosthesis with another and facilitates adjustment for length. Both methods have their places in the fabrication of prostheses.

Joints and joint mechanism

Joints have two purposes in prosthetics; the first is to replace an absent joint, the second to provide a desired range of movement in an ancillary suspensory, stabilizing or control device.

Mechanisms are devices which activate or modify joint movements. Joints may allow movement in one, two or three planes, or in no plane at all, and can be further differentiated as follows:
1 motion in one designated plane
   (a) about one axis — uniaxial
   (b) about multiple axes — polycentric
2 motion in two designated planes
   (a) about two axes — dual axis
3 motion in three planes
   (a) about finite axes — multiaxial
   (b) about an infinite number of axes — flexible
4 no motion in any plane — rigid

The term 'rigid' has been disputed by some but there are 'joints' in carpentry which are rigid, and engineers use bonding, welding and rivets. Furthermore, there are times when the natural joint is best replaced at the natural level by a prosthetic device which is rigid.

'Flexible' may be a short piece of spring, plastic or other flexible material which allows motion in three planes and is readily recognized as a joint, but long cords, straps elasticated material which are used in suspension or control are also 'flexible joints' allowing freedom of movement. When such freedom is not desired these 'joints' must be replaced with a more rigid structure easily seen to be a joint.

Joints as described above give freedom of movement in the designated planes only restricted by the inherent friction.

Joint mechanisms are used to move or modify the action of joints and the following are the types of modifications used in prosthetics.

Stops

Natural joints have their ranges of movement limited by ligaments or bony structures. To be lifelike, a prosthetic joint also needs to have the extremes of movement limited mechanically. Such mechanical stops are given names which, since there is as yet no agreed international terminology, vary worldwide. It is sufficient to recognize that most prosthetic joints require mechanisms which limit the range of movement. These 'stops' can then act as do natural ligaments in giving static stability, and to prevent excessive motion.

Locks

To give stability, and to maintain a posture, a joint may be provided with a lock. A lock when actuated prevents all movement of the joint in its designated range of motion. These are usually optional, but particularly in lower-limb prostheses for the elderly or feeble they may be automatic. Some are only operative in one position, others may act on a quadrant giving several specific positions of locking, and some others can operate at an infinite number of positions within a limited range. Most mechanisms with this function are called locks but there are mechanisms in both upper and lower limbs which go by other names. It is important to recognize whether the intention is to prevent movement in any direction when the mechanism is operating, or only to modify it.

In this connection it is worth mentioning the so-called 'ratchet lock' sometimes used in prosthetic elbow joints. This mechanism prevents extension of the elbow in a succession of positions as the elbow is flexed using a ratchet. It does not inhibit flexion. Indeed to regain full extension the elbow is first fully flexed. Such a mechanism is not in fact a lock but a variable extension stop.

Mechanisms moving joints

There are three sources of power used to move parts of a prosthesis: the body's musculature, gravity acting on the body or the prosthesis, and external power.

The body's musculature. This operates by the stump acting on the socket. It firstly moves the whole prosthesis in space in the direction that the stump moves, but where there is a freely mobile joint below the stump it will, due to inertia, cause the more distal parts of the prosthesis to rotate in a contrary direction, thus producing what is often a desired movement. Body power can also be transmitted by means of straps, cables or levers from more distant parts of the body. Such mechanisms are commonly used in the upper limb but, although common at one time, are now infrequently used in the lower limb. The kinetic energy imparted to the prosthesis and its components in this manner may then be used to store up potential energy to modify the motion.

Gravity. Gravity is a source of power which acts directly on parts of a prosthesis to give a desired movement, or by action on the prosthesis or the body's mass provides potential energy which can later be used to initiate or modify movement.

External power. The use of external power is a comparatively new development in prosthetics, which has progressed over the past three decades. Because we are considering prostheses and not mobility aids, the power source, as well as the motor, must be carried in the prosthesis or on the person. Bulk and weight of a power source have imposed limitations in the use of external power.

The lower limbs in use are active all the time, and their activity is demanding on the use of power. All levels of lower-limb amputation involving only one limb can use prostheses of current design for a satisfactory level of walking. If greater mobility is needed the amputee can use the other means of mobility which the non-amputee also uses, such as cars, elevators (lifts), escalators, etc., or powered wheelchairs.

In the upper limb much of the use of movement is intermittent; the elbow once flexed can be locked, and the gripping hand can maintain its grasp without calling on the power source until a new position is desired. Of the possible sources of power, thermopneumatic systems have not been used but might possibly be of use in the future. Electrohydraulic systems have been tried but hydraulic systems have always provided a leakage problem. Pneumatic systems were used for some years in the United Kingdom and Europe because at that time the response of pneumatic motors was faster and quieter than available electric systems, and for a time gas cylinders had better duration than battery systems. Pneumatic systems have now largely been phased out because there is no way of reducing the bulk of the gas cylinders which did not provide enough duration for reasonable levels of activity in daily life, and because electric motors and rechargeable batteries have been reduced in bulk, weight and durability. The motors have been greatly improved in efficiency and combine well with the complex electronic control systems which are now available.

Motion assisting and resisting mechanism

Compression or stretching of springs and elastomers, either by gravity or by an imparted movement, is used to provide potential energy to assist in accelerating a contrary movement, particularly in its initial stage. Such mechanisms will also resist the movement, which provides their potential energy. Such resistance is usually desirable for there is normally a need to decelerate a movement at the end of the desired range. There are also mechanisms — friction, pneumatic, hydraulic, etc. — which are used to give this deceleration without there being any corresponding reciprocal acceleration.

These assisting and resisting mechanisms are intended to correspond to the accelerations and decelerations by which the normal musculature controls the movements of the natural limb. The variation of power, timing, and duration of the action of normal musculature is highly complex and individual. The prosthetic mimicry of movement is poor although improving in the action of some artificial joints. The active person with a good amputation in the lower limb can walk on the level at a steady pace in a way which will deceive most people who are not trained observers, but the movements carried out in everyday life by the upper limb, such as eating or combing the hair, are so complex and individual that, however efficient, they are instantly recognizable as artificial.

COSMETIC COMPONENTS

Cosmetic components are those parts of a prosthesis which are used solely to satisfy the psychological loss, and are of two types. The one replaces the soft tissues of the limb and gives shape, the other provides a skin. The structure of an exoskeletal prosthesis is usually shaped to give a realistic appearance but, as its purpose is to be load-bearing, it is not a cosmetic component per se. Attempts were sometimes made to reduce the dimensions of the exoskeletal limbs to allow some soft covering, but this was rarely thick enough to give significant softening, and added weight which was usually unacceptable.

The current use of a central post to transmit the load has made use of a soft, shaped infrastructure. Various spongy materials can be used, mostly one of the foam plastic materials which can be shaped to match the normal limb and are compliant when pressed.

The 'skin' components are of different types. Firstly there are coloured enamel or matt-finished paints or coloured leather used on the surface of exoskeletal limbs. Secondly, there are shaped fairings used without an underlying soft component; made of glass fibre, nylon fibre or other similar material impregnated with plastic, they are prefabricated to standard shapes and sizes which cannot be altered. They are light shelf items giving a superficial resemblance to the natural limb which may satisfy the patient. They cannot be reshaped to give a close resemblance to the normal limb. Lastly, there are plastic covers pulled over an underlying soft shaped material which are coloured to resemble the appearance of normal skin, and which may have for the upper limb representation of superficial veins, and even hairs. These covers are expensive, although they are becoming cheaper. There are some problems with them. Firstly, with exposure to light those resembling Aryan skin gradually darken, which is acceptable as spring moves on to summer and autumn but can become unacceptable in winter. Secondly, though washable and resistant to normal dirt, printer's ink, ball-point ink, and carbon paper sink into the plastic very rapidly and cannot be removed. These covers, particularly those on artificial hands, may need to be replaced solely because of discoloration.

ALIGNMENT DEVICES

It is not the purpose of this book to act as a manual on the manufacturing techniques used in prosthetics. Alignment devices are tools used in lower-limb fabrication. They are included here solely because some are left in the prostheses as permanent fixtures.

The nature of the loading and the freedom of movement of both the natural and prosthetic joints of the upper limb make fine adjustments of the socket relative to the rest of the prostheses unnecessary.

In the lower limb a change of 1° at the hip level can make a shift of the reaction at the foot level of the order of 2–3 cm, which is of great significance relative to the axial load. Until about 1950 the prosthetist was dependent on rule of thumb and his own experience to align the prosthesis — so-called 'bench alignment'. Bench alignment is still the first step but, in recent years, a number of devices have been developed which allow adjustment of the spatial relationship of the socket relative to the foot giving shift of the socket mediolaterally and anteroposteriorly, as well as giving angular adjustments for flexion-extension, abduction-adduction, and rotation.

Those devices which are removed from the prosthesis before finishing we need not consider further, except to observe that their removal alters the distribution of mass and therefore the natural cadence of the prosthesis. Those left in have no function in the completed prosthesis unless a realignment is required.

Alignment devices may be sited at one or both ends of a limb segment and vary considerably in design (such as wedge-shaped discs, saucers, pyramidal shapes, etc.) which can be adjusted and readjusted to get the optimum alignment in both static and dynamic use. If they are not removed before completion of the prosthesis they should be fixed in position so that they do not move.

It is obvious that there are considerable gaps in the technology available to reproduce the function of a lost limb. At some levels of amputation even the principles given here cannot be fully applied, which is evident in the examples given of prostheses for the different levels of amputation in later chapters.

5

Principles of Amputation Surgery

The purpose of amputation is to remove disease or deformity. But in diseases such as diabetes or atherosclerosis for which amputation may be the treatment of choice, it is only possible to remove the local manifestation. Once this primary purpose is satisfied there is usually the desire to restore function. Occasionally this objective is approached by further surgical procedures but in the overwhelming majority of patients function is restored by means of an artificial device or prosthesis.

Without the amputation there is no prosthesis and the amputation stump is an essential part of the prosthesis, being the foundation on which the prosthesis depends.

The amount of function which can be restored by a prosthesis depends on two factors: firstly the residual function of the body as a whole and particularly of the amputation stump for the control of the device, and secondly the degree of engineering skill in the design of its components to reproduce acceptable levels of mimicry.

An understanding of the physical properties of the biological tissues, as well as the pathological state, is necessary if the adverse effects of amputation are to be kept to the minimum, while at the same time making the most of the residual functions.

Amputation involves many different tissues which may be altered not only by the amputation itself but also by the unnatural loading imposed on them by a prosthesis. Such changes can affect prosthetic design. The limitations of currently available prosthetic techniques and materials may render otherwise sound surgical procedures unsatisfactory in practice.

Voluntary movement is initiated in response to sensory input from sight, sounds, smell, feel or joint sense, whether the action is immediate or delayed. Sight and sound have a place in the management of a prosthesis, particularly of the upper limb, and are not impaired by amputation, but the major factor in the control is the sensory input from skin, muscles, ligaments, and joints.

Amputation is through skin, superficial fascia, muscles, ligaments and bone or joints. A short revue of their properties and the consequences of amputation follows.

BIOLOGICAL TISSUES AND THE EFFECTS OF AMPUTATION

Skin

Skin is a limiting membrane which prevents excessive loss of body fluids and provides a barrier to the invasion of the body by bacterial and noxious substances. It is a sense organ giving the sensation of touch, temperature and pain. It has a rich blood supply and can excrete some waste products through sebaceous and sweat glands by which it also provides an important mechanism for heat control.

It is elastic and has a grain, but its structure varies over the extensor and flexor aspects. In most areas it moves over the underlying tissues, but in some parts, such as the heels and finger pulp, it is much less mobile, being adapted together with the underlying tissues to absorb impact, loading and shear. The skin with normal sensation and with a normal vascular bed can withstand high loads applied intermittently, particularly in those adapted areas but, being dependent on the capillary pressure of its blood supply, cannot withstand constant pressures greater than 5.0 kN/m^2 applied indefinitely.

Skin is currently the component of the body through which all the forces arising at the interface between the prosthesis and body are transmitted. It is at this interface that, other than sight and hearing, sensory information is transmitted, on which the prosthetic control depends. It is important to plan the incision so that the shear effect is the least possible at the site of the incision scar. Other forces are taken as far as possible on skin adapted for load and elsewhere are distributed as widely as possible to lessen the load per unit area.

Anaesthetic areas of skin are always a potential hazard. Provided the load per unit area can be kept low such areas may sometimes be acceptable in the lower limb but should not normally be retained in the upper limb.

Superficial fascia

Between the skin and deeper tissues lies a layer of subcutaneous fat. It varies in thickness and consistency from one part of the body to another and also in individuals. It has a poor blood supply and provides thermal insulation. It permits the skin to move over the deeper structures. This introduces an element of instability because the deeper tissues can have a measure of longitudinal angular deviation, rotation, and pistoning within the enveloping skin. In the grossly obese this can complicate the use of a prosthesis.

However, it has some advantages for its compliant nature permits change in shape and volume by the active muscles, allows tolerance of the differences between complex anatomical movement and simpler prosthetic joints, and helps energy absorption under impact-loading, particularly in those areas such as the heel and finger pulp, where it is structured with the skin to do so.

Deep fascia

The deep fascia is a fibrous sheet-like structure of variable toughness which encompasses the muscles to which it may be attached, and to which it provides a flexible structural support. It is chemically allied to, and is similar in structure to, tendons and ligaments with which it sometimes merges.

Muscles

Voluntary muscles are controlled by the motor cortex and are the source of power by which purposeful movements are made. They may also act involuntarily. They have an origin which is proximal and may be multiple from ligaments, fascia and septa, as well as bone, a belly which is contractile and supplies the power, and a distal attachment by a tendon. This is normally a short structure and localized but may be long to enable the muscle power to operate remotely and, by a pulley-like action, change the direction of the force exerted.

Fibrous organs and tendons are relatively avascular and bleed little on division. Muscle bellies are highly vascular and bleed profusely. Muscle fibres forming muscle bellies exert forces by contracting in length and increasing in cross-section, thus altering the configuration. There is also an absolute change in volume, for in man the blood flow in resting muscles may be as low as 2–3 ml per 100 g/min but with activity can rise as high as 70 ml per 100 g/min. The vascular shunt through muscle reduces the blood flow through skin and bone in normal man, a switch which may have grave consequences in the dysvascular patient.

It is common to refer to all tissues that are not bone as soft tissues. The resting muscle is indeed soft and compliant but, when exerting its maximum force, can be hard and its tendon can become a rigid bar.

Muscles acting about a joint are arranged in opposite groups of agonist and antagonist to each particular movement, and in health balance each other. This state of balance is disturbed by amputation because the origins and insertions of the opposing groups are often at different levels.

Nerves

Nerves have little mechanical significance in affecting prosthetic design except that the healing process in a divided nerve produces a bulb which, if exposed to pressure or tension, can produce pain. Amputation causes a loss of sensory input impairing awareness, particularly of spatial relations on which motor control depends.

Circulatory system

Blood flows from the heart at relatively high pressures which diminish as the lesser arteries and arterioles are reached, so that blood flow entering the capillaries is at low pressure. From the capillaries it is drained into the venous system in which the pressure is in part hydrostatic. Flow in these vessels back to the heart is helped by elevation, but in large part is maintained by muscular activity and the valves in the veins. Relatively low circumferential pressures can easily impair lymphatic and venous return while having little effect on arterial flow.

A limb does not normally receive its blood supply from a single artery but from two or more principal arteries which have some intercommunication through lesser vessels. Sudden occlusion of major vessels may deprive tissues of a blood supply, leading to their death, but if the impairment is slow to develop, smaller vessels may enlarge sufficiently to provide an adequate collateral circulation. An important collateral circulation is that through the nutrient arteries of the bones, in which there is a connection through the growth plate scar between arteries entering the shafts of long bones and the circulation round the joints. As much as 20% of the normal circulation may reach the periphery by this route which can be enough to maintain viability if there is a reduced activity of the limb, or be capable of maintaining a more distal amputation if left unimpaired.

In amputation arteries diminish in bore after a long period of time because of the reduced call from the periphery.

Ligaments

Ligaments are bands or sheets of tough fibrous material which connect two or more bones or other structures and under tension can become rigid. They provide stabilizing and limiting mechanisms for joints by which much of the static posture can be maintained with little or no muscular effort. They also provide through their nerve supply sensory information about that posture.

Bone

Bone is a 'hard' material consisting of an organic matrix impregnated with mineral salts, the ratio of the two components varying from bone to bone and in different parts of the same bone. It also varies in response to health and disease and the long-term forces exerted on it. Long bones are encased, except at the joints, in a tough membrane or periosteum which has a rich network of vessels contributing to the nutrition of the bone. The periosteum is involved in the growth process and after maturity maintains the architecture, repair of fractures, etc. Bones have an external layer of dense cortical bone and internally a layer of spongy or cancellous bone. Long bones have a shaft mostly composed of cortical bone with a small amount of cancellous bone and a central core of fatty tissue, the medulla; they broaden at each end where the cortical bone becomes thinned and the cancellous bone increases, obliterating the central medullary cavity. The small bones of the wrist and ankle have only a thin layer of cortical bone enclosing cancellous bone.

Where bones articulate with each other the bone is covered with cartilage. In children the shafts of the long bones are separated from the expanded ends by epiphyseal cartilage from which growth in length takes place. With maturity this cartilage is absorbed and the epiphysis is united with the shaft but, at this site, there is a well-defined line which has a rich anastomosis between the nutrient vessels of the shaft and the circulation of the epiphysis and joint which can provide an important collateral system.

Bone has grain and can accept high loading in a preferred direction. The cortical shafts of long bones can accept high loading but, on amputation through these bones, the small cross-sectional area produces a high load per unit which the tissue covering them cannot tolerate if there is full end-bearing. The cancellous bone of the expanded ends of long bones is well adapted to tolerate impact and the larger area reduces the load per unit area which the tissues covering them can usually tolerate, particularly as these tissues are usually from those which are adapted for higher loads.

Bone can become demineralized by hormonal and vitamin deficiencies as by disease. It can also become demineralized by disuse as in paralysis or in amputation if it is not subjected to a load. Such demineralized bone can become painful.

Joints

In limbs the joints which have a significant range of movement are between bones covered by cartilage bathed by fluid excreted by the synovial membrane. Normal joints have a coefficient of friction of less than 0.002. They are moved by the action of muscles but their range is limited primarily by ligaments which also sustain many common postures. Joints have to transmit forces between bones. These forces have two components: those arising externally in performing a function, and those arising internally from muscular action. Those arising externally are from the workload, which is often in response to gravity as in supporting the body weight in standing, or carrying a load in the hand. The internal forces arise from muscular action used to maintain joint stability. These forces can be surprisingly high when leverage multiplies the forces needed. For instance, straight leg raising exerts a force between the surfaces of the hip joint which is as high as six times body weight, and a similar factor of six operates on the elbow when holding a weight in the hand with the elbow flexed at 90°.

This summary of the characteristics of the various tissues is common knowledge to medical students. They are the basis upon which good amputation techniques depend.

Whatever the cause, amputation is an unnatural state. Single amputation disturbs symmetry of the body mass, and symmetrical movement thereafter can only be achieved with a significant energy penalty. The energy potential of the body is diminished by the muscle loss and the heat-loss mechanism is lessened by the skin loss. At lower levels of amputation these changes are minimal but patients with high level or multiple amputations may have difficulty in dissipating the heat of metabolism, even when the actual metabolic rate may be abnormally low. The multiple amputee may become gross on a very restricted diet which may need vitamin additives. The peripheral loss of musculature may cause arteries to diminish in bore because of the reduced circulatory need, which with advancing years may have serious consequences. To this must be added the sensory loss which is particularly significant in the upper limb. Lastly, there is the loss of body image which can be the most serious loss of all.

Amputation is always, therefore, a skin disease, a sensory impediment, a neuromuscular condition, a skeletal deformity, a metabolic disorder, and a psychological problem. Enough has been said to show that every effort should be made to keep these consequences to the minimum and to restore as nearly as possible the normal function of the remaining tissues.

When amputating, the surgeon is providing the foundation on which the use of the prosthesis depends and so he/she should have some understanding of the limitations of current prostheses, for these may impose limitations on the surgical technique, if both are to combine to give the best available outcome.

BASIS OF SURGICAL TECHNIQUE

Guidelines can now be given on techniques common to all levels of amputation. Prostheses can be fitted to any level of amputation but some levels can so restrict the use that a less satisfactory prosthesis results.

A limb is a system of joints and levers. A prosthetic limb is not the best engineering solution to the problem; it is the best solution to the problem with similar levels of joints and levers as the natural limb.

The amputation stump is the lever which controls the prosthesis. It is inserted into a socket and must be a long enough lever to function. Retention of limb remnants below a joint which cannot move the part is rarely justified except in a few, mostly congenital, deformities when further surgery may produce a longer worthwhile stump.

Section of bone just above a joint may also be a disadvantage for it may prevent the use of the best type of artificial joint, which section a few centimetres higher would have permitted without seriously shortening the lever. New prosthetic joints have in recent years made more distal section acceptable at many levels.

Lastly, while exceptional, joints at anatomical level which are arthrodesed or ankylosed may be retained if, as may happen in severe trauma, they provide better stumps for load-bearing at a lower level than is available above the joint; otherwise ankylosed or arthrodesed joints are an embarrassment for they do not function themselves and prevent their artificial replacement from doing so. Section at joint level or above is then favoured.

There are two types of amputation: (1) through or near a joint, and (2) through the shaft of a long bone. Both have their advantages and disadvantages. Many surgeons have tried at various levels to overcome the disadvantages of the one while also trying to increase the advantages of the other, usually to the detriment of both.

These surgical modifications are often attempts to overcome real or imagined prosthetic problems which are better solved by new technical prosthetic design.

AMPUTATION THROUGH OR NEAR A JOINT (DISARTICULATION)

Advantages

1   The expanded cancellous bone, adapted to impact and load-bearing in its natural state, remains to provide end-bearing for transmission of loads through the shaft and to provide a normal pathway for proprioception from that level.
2   The skin and superficial fascia at the heel, knee, buttock and elbow have areas that are adapted to accept impact and high loads. These areas can naturally be used to cover the bone, and for the transmission of forces at the stump–socket interface.
3   In children the cartilaginous growth plate is preserved and in adults the collateral circulation from the shaft through the growth plate scar to the epiphysis is retained.
4   Few muscle bellies are divided, the section being through fibrous origins or tendinous insertion, the latter making reattachment easier.
5   The area is less vascular and control of bleeding at operation is eased, lessening the risk of complication.
6   The medullary cavity of the shaft is not opened and the risk of infection spreading is reduced.
7   The bulbous expansion provides suspension of the prosthesis and an element of rotatory control, and the long bone, preserved in its entirety, provides a long lever.
8   Stump pain is a rarity in these amputations.
These advantages must not blind us to the disadvantages common to all these amputations.

Disadvantages

1   There have been some problems in obtaining healing at some levels but these have largely been overcome in recent years by re-design of the skin flaps.
2   The destroyed joint cannot be replaced prosthetically at the same level within the dimensions of the normal limb. In the past, joints had to be placed on either side, making a wide and unsightly joint. Of recent years, at most levels joints are now

available which, although placed below the normal level, have their axis of rotation at the normal level. These are in use although there are still some problems of design, weight and durability.

3   The bulbous end prevents the proximal insertion of the stump into the socket if shapely contours are to be preserved. Either a tubular shape of a cross-section which can accept the bulbous end must be used with an inner soft section shaped to the contours to maintain adhesion, or a shaped socket with an opening at the front or side through which the stump can be laid, and then kept in place by some method of closure.

There are prosthetic problems which can make these levels unacceptable to some amputees, usually women on the grounds of appearance. Surgeons have tried from time to time to overcome them by surgical means. Basically this is by one of two ways. One is to make a section at a slightly higher level where there is a lesser cross-section. The other is to remove the bulbous sides of the epiphysis. Both reduce the cross-section of bone, damage the epiphyseal plate anastomosis, and usually result in the skin covering the end being from an area less well adapted for load-bearing, so that few can tolerate full end-bearing. To this it must be added that these procedures result more frequently in a painful stump than does disarticulation.

Recent prosthetic design has overcome many of these problems and at some levels surgical procedures have been developed which are acceptable in special cases and are discussed in the appropriate section.

AMPUTATION THROUGH THE SHAFT OF LONG BONES

Amputations through the shafts of long bones are the commonest and also have advantages and disadvantages.

Advantages

1   A useful joint above the level of amputation is preserved. A useful joint should be mobile but may be flail, and it should have a long enough stump below it to give an adequate socket fit. It should not have any major flexion deformity, particularly in the lower limb.

2   A length of long bone is retained as a lever to assist in the transmission of the workload.

Disadvantages

1   The muscle bellies are sectioned and may be very vascular. In such cases bleeding is more difficult to control at operation.

2   There is at most levels a greater disturbance of the muscular balance between agonists and antagonists.

3   Reattachment of the divided muscles is more difficult.

4   The medullary cavity of the bone is opened and so there is a greater risk of the bone becoming infected.

5   The divided bone and the soft tissues covering it may contribute to, but cannot sustain, full end-bearing, and the workload must largely be distributed at a higher level.

There is a further distinction to be made between surgery for emergency conditions of operations, such as in wartime, train accidents, etc., contaminated wounds, infection, and a planned procedure without gross infection. In the former the amputation should be at the lowest level possible, of a guillotine type, with the minimum use of foreign materials by way of sutures, and left open initially. Secondary suturing is desirable as the wound heals. At a later date a formal revision at the site of election is planned. This may not always be done for sometimes the patient may opt to continue with the healed stump rather than undergo further surgery.

For the planned amputation the principles are the same whether through the shaft of a bone or at a joint.

1   If the medullary cavity is opened sharp edges of the divided bone should be rounded off and if possible the medullary cavity closed, preferably with a periosteal flap. This helps to maintain the normal venous vascularity and prevents venous pooling.

2   Muscle remnants should be restored to their normal fibre length and alignment, being sutured to the bone as distally as possible (a process called myodesis), and over the end of the bone as a myoplasty. It is usually necessary in amputation through the shaft to tailor the muscles which may otherwise bunch, giving rise to an undesirable bulbous stump. This attachment enables those muscles originating proximally to the joint above to exert their maximum residual force, making use of the longest possible lever, and those which no longer act about a joint can contract isometrically, thus assisting in venous return. These muscles remain innervated, and if allowed to retract fully may have periods of painful contraction and jactitation. The muscles thus restored should also insulate the cut nerve endings and the bone from the prosthesis.

3   While avoiding excessive tension on the nerves at operation they should be divided as high as possible and allowed to retract into the muscle mass.

4   Both types of fascia are carefully re-sutured, the deep to restore its supportive function, and the superficial to prevent the skin becoming adherent to deep structures.

5   The skin needs careful closure to ensure as little scarring as possible. The incision should be planned so that if possible the scar is transverse to shear forces.

6

Principles of Rehabilitation

The Oxford English Dictionary's definition of rehabilitation is: 'restore to rights; restore to previous condition'. In the case of the amputee, as for all patients, the aim must be to restore him to function that is as full as possible within his environment and physical condition. For example, it should be possible to rehabilitate a 90-year-old lady, with no great medical problems other than a below-knee amputation due to peripheral vascular disease, to an independent life in her home, walking with an aid of some sort. On the other hand, a 19-year-old youth who has an above-knee amputation due to trauma should be able to return to a working life and to walk extremely well in his prosthesis with very little outward sign that he is an amputee. He will have been advised about travelling on public transport, driving his own car, and the sports that he can participate in.

The successful rehabilitation of an amputee depends on the 'complete team' approach. The professionals included in the team are: surgeon, nurses, physiotherapist, occupational therapist, social worker, psychologist, and prosthetist. It is becoming more common for a prosthetist from the local Limb-Fitting Centre to visit hospitals and attend ward rounds that include amputees as new patients. Without good communication between all these professionals successful rehabilitation is unlikely, as the patient's programme cannot be organized or monitored thoroughly enough.

Factors affecting the restoration of a degree of function in these patients are as follows:
1 mental attitude and approach
2 physical ability of the patient
3 level of amputation
4 rehabilitation programme

MENTAL ATTITUDE AND APPROACH

Amputation was formerly offered to the patient as a last resort because other treatments, such as reconstructive vascular surgery, had failed. A feeling of failure was passed on subconsciously to the patient. An amputation should therefore be offered as a positive treatment to restore the patient to better health and to an expectation of some independence. To lose a limb is a psychological trauma and after the amputation there is often a period of grieving, as after bereavement of a close relative. The amputee also has to face the fact that his body has been mutilated and is now abnormal. These feelings and problems must be recognized by the whole rehabilitation team, and the patient and his family must be helped to come to terms with them during the treatment programme and afterwards, if necessary. Often it is a great help to a patient to meet another amputee in similar circumstances and with the same level of amputation. This can be arranged either by a visit to the Limb-Fitting Centre or by asking an established amputee to visit the patient, who can benefit from talking to someone who has surmounted problems similar to his own.

PHYSICAL ABILITY OF THE PATIENT

The patient may be suffering from other medical problems, such as cardiac and pulmonary insufficiency, arthritis, hemiplegia, a confusional state, or the side-effects of chemotherapy, and this will obviously affect his ability to use a prosthesis. An assessment of the patient's abilities will determine whether wheelchair rehabilitation would be more appropriate; this again must be put to the patient as a positive treatment and not as a failure. It would be unfair to exaggerate the possible level of function after amputation as it would be to minimize it.

THE LEVEL OF AMPUTATION

The higher the level of amputation the more difficult it is to restore the patient to full functional ability, as more joints are lost and there will therefore be less muscle power to control the artificial limb. The prosthesis itself will be more complex and heavier for the higher levels of amputation. Thus the patient with a hip disarticulation cannot be as active as a patient with a below-knee amputation who has only lost one joint (the ankle), however effective the prosthesis may be. A patient who has a poor amputation at any level, which gives rise to pain and makes the prosthesis uncomfortable, will lead a less active life than if his amputation stump were good.

THE REHABILITATION PROGRAMME

The aim of the programme must be to make the best use of the remaining abilities of the patient in order to obtain the best possible level of function and to restore him to society.

If possible the programme should start preoperatively, even before the decision to amputate has been made, and should be maintained until the expected level of function has been achieved. It can be split into four stages: pre-amputation; post-amputation but pre-prosthetic; wearing temporary prosthesis; and wearing permanent prosthesis. The same general principles apply to both upper and lower limbs.

Pre-amputation stage

The patient should be assessed thoroughly at this stage and his physical state and abilities noted. The geriatric patient has probably been in pain for some time; his general condition will often be poor and would have to be improved by medication and diet. This will also ensure effective wound healing after an operation.

The patient's ability to help himself in all the activities of daily living should be assessed and noted. The physiotherapist should assess the patient's general strength and mobility. Preoperatively the physiotherapist should have noted how well the patient is able to walk, and with what footwear and aids. The surgeon should know at this stage of any flexion contractures at any joints which may affect his decision regarding the level at which to amputate. If there is more than 15° fixed flexion at the hip, a through-knee amputation should not be attempted, as that amount of flexion is not easily incorporated in the socket of the prosthesis. In such a case an above-knee amputation would result in a more cosmetic and functional prosthesis. A below-knee amputation should not be attempted if there is more than 35° fixed flexion at the knee or if the patient is hemiplegic and the limb on the affected side is to be amputated.

Once the decision to amputate has been made the rehabilitation programme must be discussed with, and explained to, the patient. It is important to explain what the patient can expect to be able to do and what will not be possible. Adjustments to his social and domestic life must be faced, and the patient will need help from staff, family, and friends in making these adjustments. It should be remembered that a young person will find it more difficult to adjust to his new body image than an elderly one.

The patient will be given a preoperative exercise programme aimed at correcting or preventing contractures and improving general strength, mobility and balance. Trunk mobility exercises will be included to help in sitting balance, rolling, moving in the sitting position, etc. The upper limbs obviously require strengthening exercises, as their strength will be essential for transfers, moving around the bed, and later for work within the parallel bars, as well as for manoeuvring a wheelchair. Due to the patient's general poor preoperative condition, the contralateral leg may be weak and resisted exercises should be given to increase power and joint range. Strength and joint range should also be improved as far as possible in the leg to be amputated.

Many patients will have been heavy smokers for many years and so preoperative breathing exercises are very important, as they may suffer from respiratory complications after an anaesthetic.

At this stage it is important to find out the patient's home conditions and if necessary to make a home visit without the patient if it is felt that he has a difficult social situation. Problems may be discovered at an early stage; solutions to those problems, or necessary housing adaptations may be got under way.

A patient who has been given adequate pain control for 48 hours preoperatively, the regime being continued for a few days postoperatively, is less likely to suffer from severe phantom sensation and pain. Advice should be given that smoking will delay healing postoperatively and could cause further problems if the patient does not stop smoking immediately.

Post-amputation but pre-prosthetic stage

The patient should return from the operating theatre with a drain and just a light fluffed gauze dressing over the suture line, both held in place with a lightly applied crêpe bandage. The dressing is taken down for the first time 2–3 days later when the drain is removed. A fresh dressing of lightly fluffed gauze is applied which is kept in place with Tubifast. This is a very light tubular dressing made by Seton Products Limited. At this stage, as has already been stated, the patient must be maintained with adequate analgesia to control his pain.

Day 1–2. For the first two days the patient will remain in the ward. The physiotherapist should maintain chest-care and treat the patient according to his individual needs. The patient should be encouraged to look at and handle the stump, as it is often very difficult for him to accept the look of it.

The exercise programme at this point consists of bed mobility exercises, bridging and moving up and down the bed, etc. — assisted active movements quickly leading to active exercises for the stump, for all muscle groups, and active and resisted work for the contralateral leg.

The occupational therapist should have lent the patient a

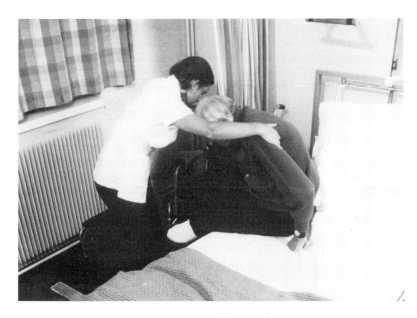

Fig. 6.1 Patient transferring into wheelchair

wheelchair until one is supplied permanently by the DHSS, if required. The patient can be taught to transfer into his wheelchair (Fig. 6.1) on the second day and before the drain has been removed. Wheelchair mobility should be taught throughout the rehabilitation programme.

Day 3 onwards. The drain is usually removed on day 3. The patient should now be able to participate in all the activities of daily living and will have a programme in the occupational therapy department. The patient should now be dressed in his clothes to attend the physiotherapy department. During the entire rehabilitation programme the amputee should travel from ward to department, etc., in his wheelchair. The stumps of all through-knee and below-knee amputees must be supported at all times by a stump board. If all the methods of oedema control are used postoperatively there should be no necessity for stump bandaging. Thus all the obvious dangers of stump bandaging are avoided.

Control of stump oedema

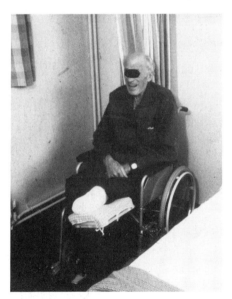

Fig. 6.2 Patient sitting in wheelchair with stump on stump-board

Wheelchair and stump board (Fig. 6.2). If a primary amputee is allowed to hop around with crutches or a frame too frequently then the stump will obviously swell, with gravity accentuating it. An oedematous stump will lead to a delay in healing, possible infection, and stump breakdown, with increased scar tissue and at the least, an ill-fitting prosthesis. Of course it is necessary for a patient to be taught safe crutch walking to enable him to get to the toilet at night, for example. This means that unless the patient is wearing a prosthesis of some sort he should travel around in a wheelchair — this applies equally to the young traumatic below-knee amputee.

The muscle pump. The below-knee amputee should be taught to contract his muscles to re-establish the peripheral vascular muscle-pump in the stump. These exercises are included in the physiotherapy exercise regime.

Pneumatic post-amputation mobility aid (PPAM aid). This has proved to be an invaluable piece of equipment for both patient and therapist (Fig. 6.3).

The equipment consists of a large plastic bag to cover the stump and a small bag, which should be invaginated, to go over the end of the stump. A metal frame encases the large bag and a pump is used to inflate it. There are two designs for the large bag: one for the above-knee amputation and one for the below-knee and through-knee amputations.

It must be remembered that this is only a partial-weight-bearing prosthesis which must only be used within parallel bars or with crutches if the patient's balance is good (Fig. 6.4).

The appropriate times of usage of the PPAM aid are as follows:
(a) The vascular amputee should be able to use the PPAM aid between 5 and 10 days postoperatively. The aid should be

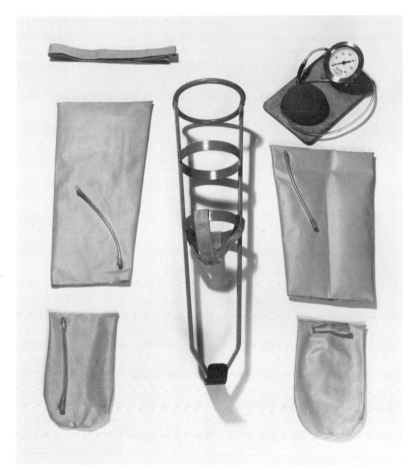

Fig. 6.3 PPAM aid equipment. From *Physiotherapy for Amputees (The Roehampton Approach)* by B. Engstrom and C. Van de Ven. Reproduced by kind permission of Churchill Livingstone.

applied over the dressings. For men the trousers can be neatly folded around the end of the stump. Jeans should be rolled back, as the seams are rather thick.

(b) The traumatic amputee may use the PPAM aid, at the surgeon's discretion, at around four days after surgery.

(c) Patients who have just had a retrim of their stump have been able to start using the PPAM aid at three days.

Advantages.
1   The main advantage is that the alternating pressure around the stump when taking a step controls the stump oedema.
2   It is the first prosthesis to 'touch' the patient's stump, and amputees begin to accept it very early on.
3   As the patient is upright and walking, his balance and gait can be re-educated right from the start.

Application. On the first day the patient may only stand in the PPAM aid and become used to the feel of the air pressure around the stump. The pressures should be between 30 and 40 mmHg. By the third day the patient should be able to wear the PPAM aid

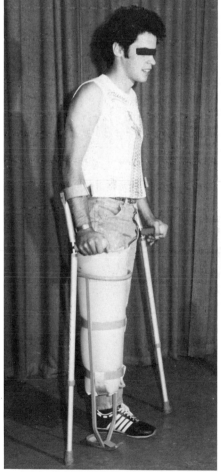

Fig. 6.4   Patient walking in the PPAM aid

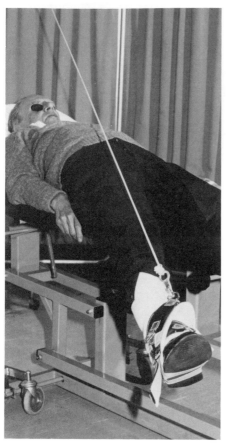

Fig. 6.5 Patient using pulleys to maintain strength of remaining leg

continuously for up to two hours. The aid should be supported when the patient is sitting and resting. It must be remembered that each patient is an individual and some suture lines heal faster than others. If a suture line is 'soggy' the aid should be removed after each walk as the line will become more moist in a hot plastic bag. Other patients may need the prosthesis to be deflated after each walk for the first two or three days. Over the past 10 years no damage has been caused to any stump while using the PPAM aid at Roehampton, as each patient is carefully supervised according to his individual needs.

When a patient has a short above-knee stump or is of tall stature it may be found necessary to use a shoulder strap to support the aid. It is also extremely inadvisable to use two PPAM aids simultaneously on bilateral amputees as it would be difficult to partial weight-bear on two legs at the same time!

Controlled environment treatment unit (CET). This technique, which was developed at Roehampton, is especially useful with lower-limb amputees. No dressings are applied, but the stump is placed in a clear plastic bag to which an air hose is attached which delivers filtered warm dry sterile air at an alternating raised pressure. The bag is kept in place with a retention harness. The CET equipment is an active wound management system enabling the surgeon to select and maintain an appropriate environment around the healing stump (see Redhead and Snowdon, 1978).

Immediate postoperative fitting of prosthesis. In some centres an immediate postoperative fitting of a prosthesis is applied immediately after amputation. Plaster of Paris is applied over the dressing which incorporates an aluminium fitting to which a simple alignment unit is attached to enable the patient to stand within 24 hours. There are obvious dangers and difficulties with this technique.
1 The suture line and wound is not visible and therefore cannot be monitored to see that it is healing correctly.
2 The plaster of Paris can easily be put on too tightly thus constricting the stump and causing a possible breakdown and necrosis of tissue, as well as causing pain.
3 The wound will be encased in a warm, moist atmosphere which is a very satisfactory medium for infection.
It has the advantage of early gait training, but now that patients can be mobilized early and with safety using the PPAM aid, the latter is the preferred method of management.

Physiotherapy programme

Assessment continues daily as part of the treatment. Treatment should be adjusted and progressed accordingly. The patient will now be attending the physiotherapy department for his treatment and he will be wearing his ordinary clothes.

1   The treatment will consist of teaching safe transfers from bed to chair and back or on to a plinth.
2   Muscle-strengthening exercises (Fig. 6.5) will be given for the arms, trunk, and normal leg.
3   Stump muscles will be strengthened by activities on the mat and bed (Fig. 6.6). Without a strong stump the patient will have little control over his prosthesis.
4   The range of movement of all joints should be maintained and increased. The patient will be advised to lie prone twice a day for at least half an hour if he is comfortable in that position. This will help to prevent contractures at the hip. It is very important to prevent contractures at the hip or knee joints so that a comfortable and cosmetic prosthesis may be applied.
5   Re-education of balance is necessary (Fig. 6.7).
6   The patient must also be advised on care of the remaining leg and foot. Only a chiropodist should care for his toe-nails, which should not be cut with scissors. Tight socks, pop socks or tights should not be worn so that any constriction is avoided.

Temporary prosthesis

The referral form to the Limb-Fitting Centre should be sent as near to the day of the patient's amputation as possible. It will take about three weeks for an appointment to be arranged, and this will coincide nicely with sutures being removed at 21 days.

Ideally the patient should remain in hospital to continue his programme on his temporary prosthesis (pylon) and only be discharged when he is independent with an aid of some kind. This is not always possible in an acute hospital, but the patient must be kept on as an outpatient in the physiotherapy and occupational therapy departments to continue his rehabilitation programme.

Fig. 6.6 Physiotherapist giving stump-strengthening exercises

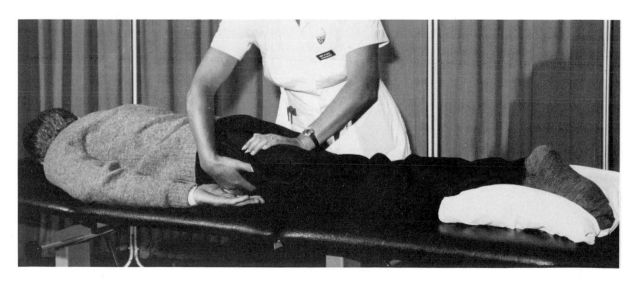

Fig. 6.7   Patient performing a balance exercise using a medicine ball

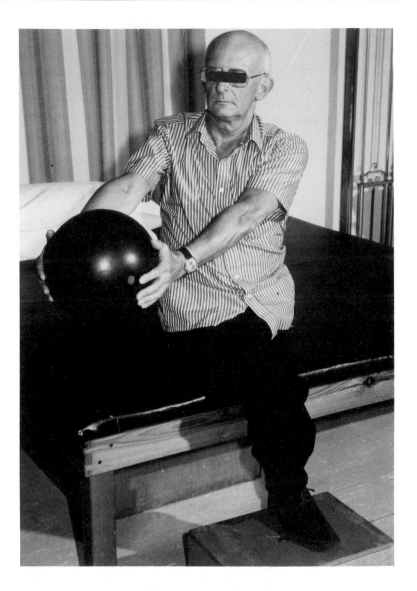

The patient's first visit to the Limb-Fitting Centre must also be discussed with him. Most patients find this a very worrying experience as no-one has told them what to expect. It should be made clear that on his first visit the patient will meet a nurse who will remove any dressings and a doctor who will view the stump and prescribe a temporary artificial leg if the stump is in good condition. The patient will then meet the prosthetist who will measure or cast for the prescribed prosthesis (pylon). That is all that is done on the first visit. The patient will be called back for a fitting of the temporary prosthesis to check that it is comfortable, and the patient will return for a third visit to take delivery of the finished pylon. The amputee should continue his rehabilitation programme using the pylon in the physiotherapy department.

The aims of the treatment will be to:

1   stand and transmit body weight through the prosthesis
2   control the prosthesis and establish a good gait pattern
3   assess the degree of function to be obtained

The wearing of the prosthesis will also help further to reduce postoperative oedema, by the mechanical pressure of the socket and the active use of the muscles. If any flexion contractures remain, they may also be overcome by the activity.

Gait training

Gait training should start in the parallel bars (Fig. 6.8) and, once a good gait pattern has been established, a walking aid should be supplied. Crutches and frames should be avoided if possible. Sticks, tripods, or a combination are best and give the patient more independence.

During this period the patient must learn to understand his prosthesis, and this should also be explained to relatives, who

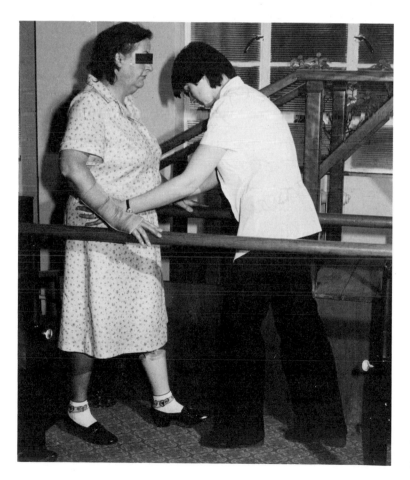

Fig. 6.8 Walking with pylon in parallel bars. Reproduced from *Cash's Textbook of General Medical and Surgical Conditions for Physiotherapists* (Downie P.A. ed.) by permission of the publishers, Faber and Faber

should be invited to visit the department during a treatment period. The patient should be able to put on and take off the prosthesis independently, to sit and stand safely, walk correctly, and manage stairs, kerbs, and slopes. If the patient is fit enough to manage transport he should be escorted on a journey, taught to manage escalators, and how to get in and out of a car. As it is possible that the patient might at some time have a fall, he must be taught how to get up from lying.

Home assessment

While the amputee is still in the early stages of rehabilitation, and before being discharged from hospital, a home visit will be arranged. The visit should be made by the physiotherapist, occupational therapist, and social worker together. A visit without the patient may be necessary at first, if there are social problems, to get an idea of what aids and adaptations will be necessary, i.e. wheelchair ramps, door-widening, handrails, or raised toilet seats, etc. A follow-up home visit can then be arranged with the patient and his relatives (Fig. 6.9). The occupational therapist will arrange for any further adaptations that are necessary, while the physiotherapist will help the patient to overcome any physical problems encountered. The social worker

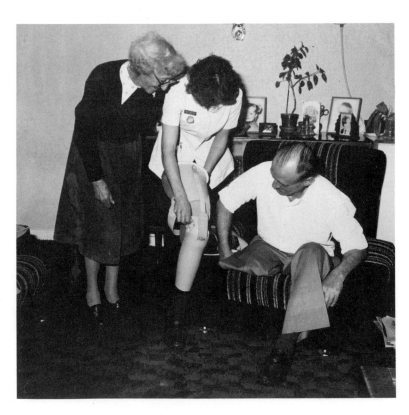

Fig. 6.9 On the home visit the artificial leg must also be explained to the relatives

will arrange any social services considered necessary, i.e. meals-on-wheels, or home help, so that all is prepared for the patient's homecoming.

Permanent prosthesis

The patient will have been discharged home and will have been using his pylon for a few weeks or months before he is measured for his definitive prosthesis. The time scale will differ for each individual: some patients, e.g. a geriatric patient suffering from diabetes may have a stump that takes longer to stabilize than others. A young traumatic amputee will probably have a stump that will settle in a matter of a few weeks. The final stage of rehabilitation is reached when the patient receives his definitive prosthesis. This is often a more complex artificial limb but is cosmetically more acceptable than the pylon.

Fig. 6.10 A double above-knee amputee, wearing short rocker pylons, learning to climb stairs

Fig. 6.11 A double above-knee amputee wearing definitive prostheses having to lean well forward to attempt a slope. From *Physiotherapy for Amputees (The Roehampton Approach)* by B. Engstrom and C. Van de Ven. Reproduced by kind permission of the publishers, Churchill Livingstone.

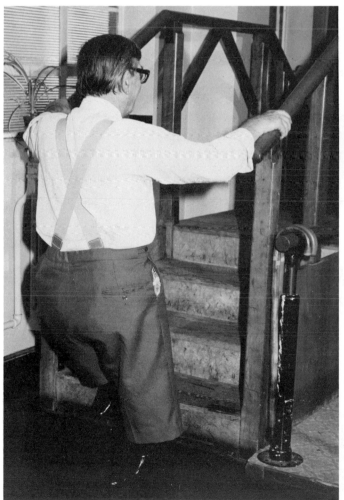

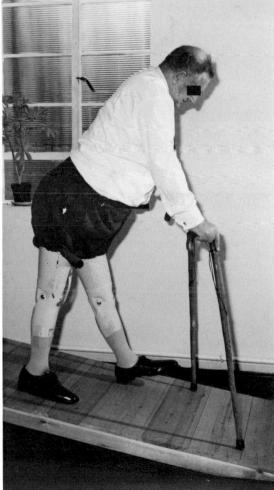

6.10

6.11

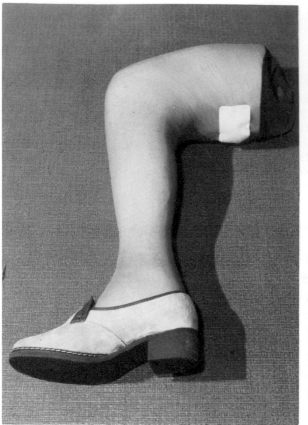

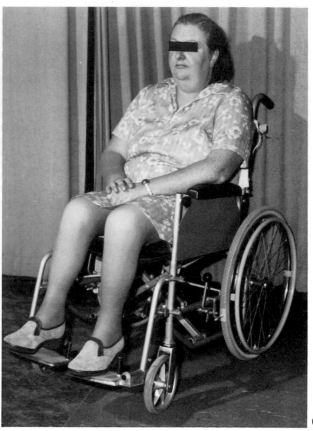

(a)

(b)

Fig. 6.12 (a) An above-knee cosmetic prosthesis. (b) A double above-knee amputee wearing cosmetic prostheses in her wheel-chair. Both (a) and (b) are from *Physiotherapy for Amputees (The Roehampton Approach)* by B. Engstrom and C. Van de Ven. They are reproduced by kind permission of Churchill Livingstone.

Training with the permanent prosthesis is a continuation of training with the pylon. Attention must be given to the gait pattern, as bad gait habits, once acquired, are very difficult to eradicate. The younger patient should make great efforts to walk with as normal a gait as possible. This would prevent postural problems occurring later in life. The older person should be satisfied with a less normal gait if he can move independently, in comfort, and within his physical capacity.

Bilateral amputee

The rehabilitation programme for the bilateral amputee is the same as for a single amputee, with the emphasis placed on balance, arm strength, and prevention of contractures.

A double amputee with two below-knee amputations is more likely to be successfully rehabilitated with his prostheses than one with two above-knee amputations, or with one above-knee and one below-knee: the higher the level of amputation, the greater the expenditure of energy required to walk. Although double above-knee amputees may find the effort required to walk with prostheses too great, all such patients should have the opportunity to make the attempt, using pylons, so that they may make the decision themselves whether or not to continue. If they do discard their prostheses, they should be offered cosmetic non-weight-bearing pylons (Figs 6.12a,b) to wear for social use.

A double amputee who lost one leg much earlier and has already walked very well with one prosthesis is more likely to be successfully rehabilitated with two prostheses in the long-term, particularly if both amputations are below knee. Once his balance, transfer, and wheelchair manoeuvres are adequate, the double amputee will need to practise activities of daily living with the occupational therapist; this will include dressing on the bed, toilet transfers, bathing, cooking, and washing from a wheelchair. These patients must be accomplished at all wheelchair manoeuvres, and be able to transfer to and from a car using a sliding board if necessary.

The patient should be followed up at home by members of the rehabilitation team between one and three months after discharge from hospital to ensure that he is coping successfully.

7

Amputation and Vascular Disease

In vascular disease amputation may be required to save life, but more often it is required to restore function when this has been lost from ischaemia.

While surgery may be effective in restoring blood supply to an ischaemic leg, this is not always so. The pain from anoxic tissue is usually underestimated and it can rapidly lead to mental deterioration, sleep loss, and anorexia, which pave the way for bronchopneumonia and renal insufficiency. Ischaemia can therefore be enough to cause death without any other factor. In addition, infection of gangrenous tissues may lead to bacteraemia or septicaemia and the toxic effects can be severe; a special risk is run by diabetics in whom invasion by anaerobic organisms, including Clostridia, can quickly be lethal. In these circumstances removal of gangrenous tissue by amputation will save the patient's life, but it is often forgotten that the amputation can be the means of the patient's rehabilitation provided that the amputation contributes, with a prosthesis, to the formation of a new organ of locomotion.

Ischaemic disease is responsible for nearly 80% of all lower-

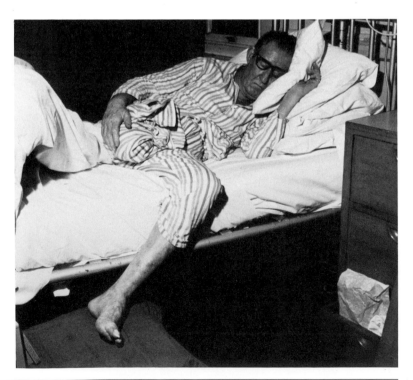

Fig. 7.1 Nocturnal rest pain of vascular origin, partly relieved by hanging the foot out of bed in the cold

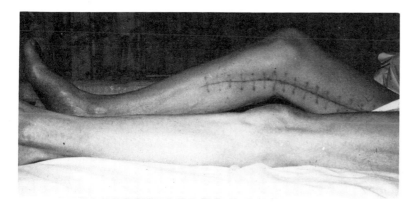

Fig. 7.2 Flexion contractures following arterial surgery

limb amputations; with the exception of a small group of younger patients with thrombo-angiitis obliterans, these are all elderly patients who pose serious problems in management and rehabilitation. The conditions responsible for limb ischaemia will be considered — acute vascular disorders first and then chronic vascular diseases.

ACUTE VASCULAR CONDITIONS LEADING TO AMPUTATION

Acute arterial occlusion and, less commonly, acute venous occlusion can cause peripheral ischaemia sufficient to require an amputation. It is well to remember that acute ischaemia with swelling of the limb is likely to be venous in origin, unless the leg has been held dependent for long periods to relieve ischaemic pain, where a venous thrombosis may be added.

Fig. 7.3 Dry painless digital gangrene. Separation may occur without the need for amputation of the digits. Walking in a suitable shoe is encouraged

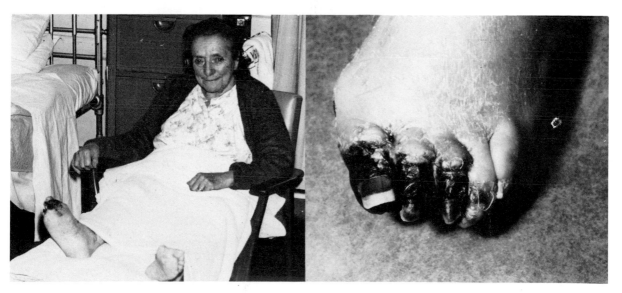

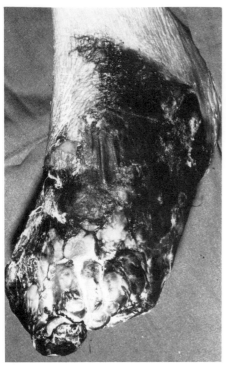

Fig. 7.4 Mummification in neglected dry gangrene

Venous gangrene

Venous gangrene associated with an iliac vein thrombosis was rarely seen even when phlegmasia cerulea dolens — the swollen cyanosed cold leg seen in this condition — was not treated effectively. With the development of more effective thrombolytic agents, such as streptokinase, urokinase, and ancrod, conservative treatment has improved on the results of heparin and anticoagulants used previously. Although the late results of emergency venous thrombectomy are not significantly better than those of conservative treatment, where venous gangrene is threatened emergency venous thrombectomy has the best chance of averting tissue loss. By these means the need for amputation in acute venous problems should be minimized. Where frank gangrene does occur, amputation should be delayed until a clear line of demarcation is shown. Venous gangrene is liable to become wet and care must be taken to avoid damage or infection of the necrotic tissue. Elevation of the limb by 5 to 10° and exposure in cool conditions are recommended until the time for amputation.

Acute arterial ischaemia

This results from embolism or thrombosis in a major limb artery. Thrombosis due to trauma should be recognized at the time of injury and confirmed by emergency arteriography or direct operative exploration of the damaged vessel. In this way, traumatic gangrene should be prevented in all but the most destructive injuries. Where so-called 'arterial spasm' is diagnosed, thrombosis due to contusion and internal disruption of the intimal lining

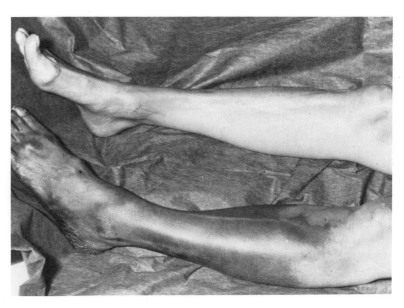

Fig. 7.5 Too late for embolectomy. Ischaemia extending to the knee, which required above-knee amputation

of the artery should be suspected. Arteriography or exploration will detect this complication and reconstruction can then be performed before irretrievable changes have occurred in the distal part of the limb.

Spontaneous arterial thrombosis is rarely seen in patients with normal blood vessels and normal circulating blood. However, it is frequently an episode in the course of chronic obliterative arterial disease and will be considered in this context. Hypercoagulability states rarely result in arterial thrombosis but may be a contributory factor.

Arterial embolism

Arterial embolism is responsible for acute limb ischaemia in patients who often have an otherwise normal peripheral vascular system. The emboli may be formed on the endothelial surface of a myocardial infarction, on the walls of the left atrium in mitral valve disease and atrial myxoma, or on the cusps of diseased aortic valves; they may also occur on the roughened plaques of aortic atheroma or in the sac of an aortic aneurysm. Paradoxical embolus rarely occurs through an atrial septal defect.

Over 80% of acute arterial emboli can be removed by operation. Most emboli at or below the aortic bifurcation can be extracted by means of a Fogarty balloon embolectomy catheter using an arteriotomy in the groin; the procedure can be performed under local anaesthetic. Even if the cardiac lesions which caused the embolus are severe, embolectomy by this means is less disturbing to the patient than any subsequent amputation that might be necessary if the patient is treated conservatively. The embolus can also be removed by arteriotomy over the embolus.

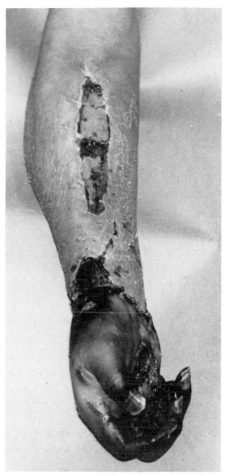

Fig. 7.6 Too late for embolectomy. Gangrene of the hand after removal of a week-old embolus from the brachial artery. The fasciotomy incision is covered by a split-skin graft.

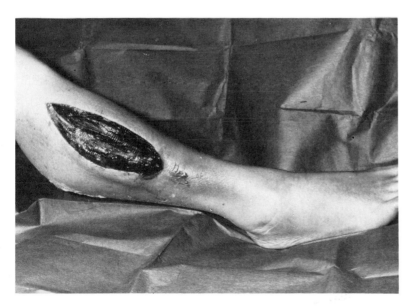

Fig. 7.7 Fasciotomy to release muscle swollen in a closed compartment

If embolectomy fails, however, amputation is required through the most distal tissue that has an adequate blood supply. Where an embolus involves an artery with atheromatous disease, or if the limb has been neglected and the patient presents with distal gangrene, the chance of re-establishing the flow is much reduced. An interval of 48 to 72 hours is sufficient to define the line of demarcation by colour and temperature. The level of amputation selected is the most distal above this line; delay is unlikely to produce a lower level of amputation. As most patients have pre-existing heart disease many are likely to be incapable of walking training with a prosthesis, but it is impossible to make a general rule and each patient must be assessed strictly on his own capabilities and cardiac state and not condemned to a wheelchair without good reason.

CHRONIC VASCULAR CONDITIONS LEADING TO AMPUTATION

Chronic obliterative arterial disease is responsible for most lower-limb amputations and is due to the deposition of atheroma which may be accompanied by medial coat sclerosis, fibrosis or calcification. Thrombo-angiitis obliterans (Buerger's disease) and diabetes mellitus also contribute to the problem.

Thrombo-angiitis obliterans

Thrombo-angiitis obliterans is a specific disease accounting for 7% of cases of obliterative arterial disease in patients under the age of 50. This disorder occurs in men in their third and fourth decade who smoke tobacco and it is characterized by multiple segmental lesions affecting both arteries and veins and causing intermittent claudication or digital gangrene which is accompanied by superficial phlebitis in most cases. This segmental pattern of occlusion and the involvement of large and small major arteries rarely permits disobliteration or bypass. Lumbar sympathectomy is of some value but unless the patient abandons his tobacco he will usually progress to a major amputation.

The level of amputation is determined by the amount of ischaemia and the lowest amputation that can be performed through normally perfused tissue is chosen. The possibility of later contralateral amputation must be considered. As these patients are otherwise young and healthy, rehabilitation is rarely a problem.

Diabetes mellitus

Diabetes mellitus is responsible for one-third of the major amputations for ischaemic disorders. The mechanisms of diabetic gangrene are complex and management is governed by the varying factors in each patient. These are:

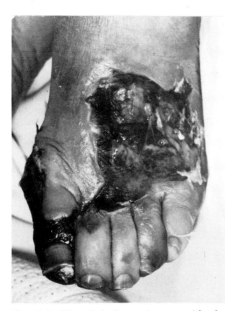

Fig. 7.8 Wet diabetic gangrene, with the ever-present risk of septicaemia and loss of diabetic control

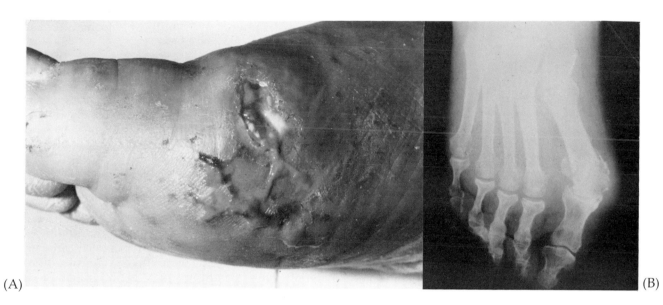

(A)   (B)

1 diffuse small vessel angiopathy
2 atheroma of major arteries
3 susceptibility to bacterial invasion due to hyperglycaemia and immunological defect
4 peripheral neuritis resulting in cutaneous trophic changes.

Fig. 7.9 Infected bunion in a patient with diabetes and arterial ischaemia. A, the outward appearance indicates deep infection in the joints, bones and deep muscle layers. B, an X-ray reveals myo-artherosis and osteomyelitis of the metatarsal

The treatment of each patient is preceded by an assessment of these factors, any or all of which may be present.

In general the diabetes must be controlled and the presence of sepsis will necessitate alteration of insulin dosage. During the acute phase continuous insulin infusion is the best method of administration. Bacterial infection must be countered by antibiotics. Anaerobic organisms, both clostridial species and streptococci, may be present requiring the use of metronidazole, but the development of deep abscesses must be detected and surgical drainage provided. Septic arthritis and osteomyelitis in the foot may not be detected without X-rays. Dramatic improvement may result from these measures and the only amputation likely to be required at this stage, when large vessel occlusion is not present, is the removal of a toe or a metatarsal 'ray' amputation to eliminate dead tissue and provide free drainage.

This situation may be seen in diabetics of any age, but elderly and 'long-duration' diabetics are more likely to have the additional problem of peripheral neuritis and large vessel disease; these contribute to more severe changes and rapidly progress to extensive gangrene which requires a major amputation.

Where major vessel occlusion is present the local infection should be controlled and arteriography will determine whether a remediable blockage is present. If this is so, a disobliteration, a profundaplasty, or a bypass procedure will be useful in restoring the blood flow and this will lessen the chance of a major amputation. When vessels below the knee are occluded a lumbar

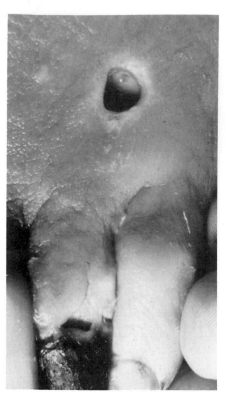

Fig. 7.10 An unusual perforating ulcer in diabetes, on the dorsum of the foot

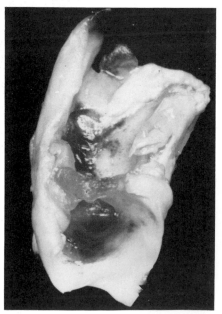

Fig. 7.11 Atheroma. An avascular stenosis removed from the common iliac artery

sympathetic block with phenol-in-Myodil, or a formal lumbar sympathectomy operation, may be of value.

While a local amputation in the presence of a major arterial block is unlikely to succeed, a major amputation can often be avoided in other groups of patients. Partial foot amputation and Syme's amputation may succeed where the vascular supply is normal. The level of amputation is determined solely by the vascular state of the tissues, provided the diabetes is stable and infection is controlled. It is therefore unwise to formulate any rule of thumb for the level of amputation in diabetics.

Arteriosclerosis

This term has been used since 1833 for chronic obliterative arterial disease and includes medial hyperplastic sclerosis (hardening of the arteries), Monkeberg's sclerosis with extensive calcification in the vessel walls, and atheroma (the subintimal accumulation of cholesterol material). These conditions may be present singly or together in any one patient.

It is important to realize that arteriosclerosis is a systemic affection and that the patient with claudication may also have angina pectoris, transient hemiplegia, abdominal pain, hypertension, or other manifestions of the disease.

The general nature of the involvement of the arteries in the individual patient is reflected in the expectation that 25 to 50% of amputees with ischaemic disease will be dead within two years and between 50 and 75% will be dead in five years (Warren and Kihn, 1968; Kihn, Warren and Beebe, 1972). Similarly 20% can expect to lose the opposite limb within two years and 33% will lose it within five years. This should be borne in mind when the factors which decide the level of amputation are considered. Only 10 to 20% of elderly bilateral amputees can be expected to walk with two prostheses and very few indeed of those with bilateral above-knee amputations.

The effects of arteriosclerosis on the lower limbs are intermittent claudication followed by ischaemic ulceration and, eventually, rest pain and peripheral gangrene. Intermittent claudication itself is an indication not for amputation but for investigation and arterial reconstruction if the patient's way of life is affected by the condition. However, ischaemic ulceration and rest pain are the warning signs of peripheral gangrene and demand investigation. A considerable amount of information can be obtained by non-invasive investigations, Doppler ultrasound, ankle systolic pressure measurements, velocity and pressure profiles at thigh, knee, and ankle levels. Arteriography shows whether arterial flow can be restored and indicates the procedure that is required. At the time of arteriography those lesions that can be dilated by balloon catheter (Gruntzig) under image-intensifier control, pressure monitoring, and the technique developed by Dotter, can be effectively treated by balloon angioplasty. This may allow revascularization without surgical intervention. The procedure

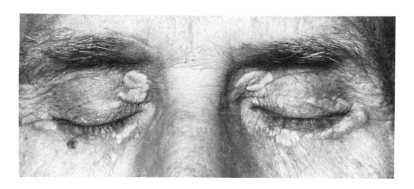

Fig. 7.12 Xanthoma palpebrarum: evidence of cholesterol deposition in extravascular sites

may also be combined with surgery at other levels to overcome the arterial occlusions and to reduce the severity and extent of the surgical treatment.

Aortic block

Required balloon angioplasty or thrombo-endarterectomy, graft bypass

Iliac block

For localized segment: balloon angioplasty. For extensive involvement: graft bypass

Femoral artery block

Single: proximal occlusion, balloon angioplasty. Long or multiple occlusion: reversed saphenous vein bypass graft or vein substitute graft or profundaplasty, balloon angioplasty

Popliteal artery occlusion

Femorodistal bypass

Tibial and distal artery block

Lumbar sympathectomy. Femorotibial bypass graft, reversed saphenous vein or substitute graft

Glutaraldehyde-treated reinforced human umbilical vein (Dardik) is the most successful vein substitute, although expensive. Polytetraflouroethylene tube (Gortex) grafts are also good vein substitutes and these have enormously increased the scope of limb-salvage operations, together with their use to provide extra-anatomical bypass grafts, e.g. axillobifemoral or femorofemoral routes to obtain revascularization. The best results of these procedures claim a 75% success rate. In the salvage of ischaemic extremities, 45 to 50% of patients with pregangrenous limbs may

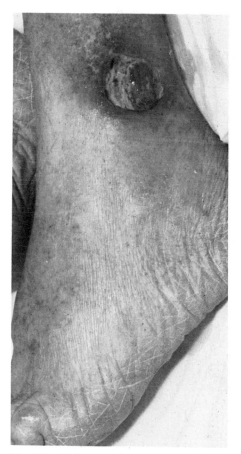

Fig. 7.13 Ischaemic ulcer at the ankle due to femoral artery occlusion in the absence of venous disorder

avoid amputation. If an arterial procedure is performed, it is often not appreciated that a femoropopliteal bypass procedure is better tolerated by a frail patient than an amputation, and a single iliac balloon angioplasty may restore flow to the profunda femoris artery and preserve the foot, even in very elderly patients. Therefore it is recommended that no patient should have an amputation without prior arteriography and the opportunity of a simple restorative procedure. It is certain that no elderly patient should have an elaborate or hazardous arterial procedure, nor should he have an arterial procedure 'to see what happens', if there is any doubt about the success of the procedure or if patency is likely to be of less than one year's duration. In this case, early amputation will give the better chance of recovery and rehabilitation.

For amputation and rehabilitation to be successful in the elderly arteriosclerotic patient, assessment should be carried out as soon as rest pain develops. The patient must not be allowed to stay in bed taking large doses of analgesics until he is a demoralized morphine addict with flexion contractures of his wasted limbs. The rest pain of ischaemic tissues is very severe and soon destroys the patient's morale which may never thereafter be restored. It is only humane to eliminate the pain by early arterial surgery or amputation. The further attrition of the patient's morale that occurs after an unsuccessful vascular procedure should be avoided by very carefully selecting patients for reconstructive operations. It is doubtful if it is ever justified to do a procedure to obtain a lower level of amputation, but a lumbar sympathectomy or sympathetic block may be combined with the amputation procedure with advantage.

INDICATIONS FOR AMPUTATION

There are two indications for amputation: (1) to remove ischaemic tissue which cannot be revascularized; and (2) to remove tissue which remains ischaemic after the blood flow has been restored (e.g. the amputation of digits or metatarsals at the time of a vascular procedure or within 10 days of it).

The indication for amputation in chronic obliterative arterial disease is thus the development of rest pain or tissue loss that cannot be reversed by vascular surgical procedures. That is, where the procedure has failed, or arteriography shows occlusion of the vessels below the popliteal artery, or an inadequate run-off prohibits reconstruction. In frail patients painless dry gangrene of small areas can be accepted provided it is certain that there is no rest pain.

Where the onset of rest pain is acute, the cause is usually to be found in a thrombosis of a segment of major artery already the seat of atheromatous disease. Often this is in the femoral artery at the level of the adductor magnus tendon, but frequently the thrombus involves the whole popliteal artery and its major

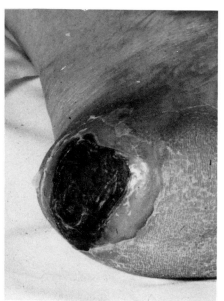

Fig. 7.14 Pressure-determined necrosis of full-thickness heel skin. This is the absolute contraindication to a Syme's amputation and a complication that must always be prevented in the patient's remaining limb

branches. If the opportunity to remove this is missed, amputation may become inevitable. Therefore patients with acute onset of rest pain should have immediate arteriography, but if this is not practicable emergency exploration of the popliteal artery will be necessary. After five days the thrombus is organized and, as propagated thrombus cannot be cleared from side branches of the distal arteries, lasting restoration of flow in the vessel is unlikely, although improvement may be obtained with a profundaplasty.

Other chronic conditions which occasionally require amputation are the unusual conditions of congenital and multiple arteriovenous fistulae, which defy correction and lead to an overgrown limb with ischaemic changes in the foot; when ulceration of the foot and necrosis of toes become intolerable, amputation restores function and activity. Similarly a deformed and hypersensitive extremity after frostbite may need amputation years later.

Venous ulceration at the ankle due to occlusion of the deep veins of the leg and incompetent lower-leg perforating veins is rarely treated by amputation, although many patients who tolerate gross incapacity and morbidity from this condition would be rejuvenated by a below-knee amputation with a modern prosthesis. Our patients in this group proved to have some of the best results in terms of achievement and quality of life after amputation. However, the most disabled patients will shrink from this treatment and many surgeons would be reluctant to advise such drastic treatment.

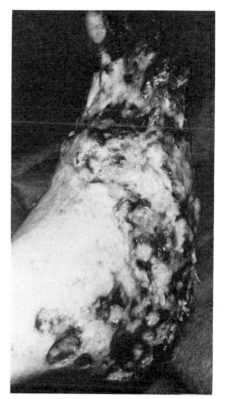

Fig. 7.15 Specific arteritis. Rheumatoid arteritis of the foot resulting in bilateral below-knee amputation

LEVEL OF AMPUTATION

The level at which amputation should be performed in obliterative arterial disease is controversial. The factors of early healing directly oppose the considerations of rehabilitation which are largely associated with the length of the amputation stump. In order to heal at all, the tissues must have an adequate blood supply and it is recommended that amputation should be performed below the most distal palpable arterial pulse to be sure of uncomplicated wound healing.

If uncomplicated primary healing is the first consideration then the majority of patients will require an above-knee amputation.

Table 7.1 Results (%) of above- and below-knee amputations in 453 patients with vascular disease

Level of amputation	Mortality	Healing		Walking
		Primary	Ultimate	
Below-knee	10	49	68	76
Above-knee	28	71	81	46

After Warren and Kihn (1968). A high proportion of above-knee amputations were performed at this time

Table 7.2a Lower limb amputations performed at Queen Mary's Hospital, Roehampton, Oct. 1974–1975

Level of amputation	Number	Percentage of total
Hind quarter	3	0.5
Hip disarticulation	14	2.2
Above knee	159	25
Gritti–Stokes	4	0.6
Through knee	115	18
Below knee	306	48
Syme's	8	1.2
Part foot	23	3.6
Total	632	

Table 7.2b Lower limb amputations performed in vascular patients at Queen Mary's Hospital, Roehampton, Oct. 1974–1975

Level of amputation	Number	Walking	Mortality
Hip disarticulation	10	5 (50%)	2 (20%)
Above knee	133	68 (51%)	12 (9%)
Gritti–Stokes	2	2 (100%)	0
Through knee	109	44 (40%)	14 (12.8%)
Below knee	256	206 (81%)	21 (8.2%)
Syme's	3	0	0
Total	513	325	49

In an analysis of 453 cases, Warren and Kihn (1968) made a comparison between the levels of amputation in ischaemic disease (Table 7.1). Ignoring differences of mortality, which probably reflect the severity of arterial disease, Fig 7.2 shows that rehabilitation to independent walking is opposed to the chance of primary wound healing. Other levels of amputation can be considered in an attempt to find the best compromise.

In the hands of an experienced surgeon, interested in the problem, satisfactory results can be obtained at all these levels of amputation (Table 7.2). The role of a major vascular procedure to achieve a lower level of amputation remains controversial. Certainly less invasive procedures such as balloon angioplasty are fully justified to achieve this purpose.

Below-knee amputation is recommended as the most frail elderly patient can be rehabilitated using a light-weight patellar-tendon-bearing or patellar-tendon-suspended below-knee prosthesis; should the patient become a double amputee an elderly patient can manage to walk with two patellar-tendon-bearing below-knee prostheses. To walk with two above-knee prostheses is a considerable achievement even for the healthy younger patient. If the elderly patient is unable to wear bilateral above-knee prostheses he has a considerable problem. He has great difficulty in rolling over in bed and, unless he has developed great strength in his arms, assistance is needed for toilet and other basic activities. His remaining mobility is provided by a wheelchair.

Intermediate levels of amputation provide a long stump which improves the ability of the patient to roll over and transfer from chair to toilet and from chair to bath, but the prostheses which must be fitted to these amputations require a full thigh socket and usually ischial tuberosity weight-bearing. The thigh socket often has lacing which many old people are unable to tie tightly enough to provide secure fitting of the prosthesis. In contrast, the patellar-tendon-bearing prosthesis is applied like a sock and requires only one buckle to secure it in position. Therefore the advantage to the patient of a below-knee stump is overwhelming, whether the amputation is unilateral or bilateral, and to achieve healing at this level the surgical technique must be modified to

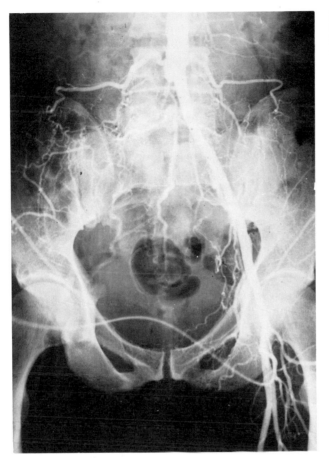

Fig. 7.16   Trans-femoral aortogram showing aortic thrombosis leading to bilateral amputation. A collateral supply usually prevents distal gangrene

give the greatest opportunity of primary healing in the presence of minimum blood supply.

In all cases preoperative preparation should include the following: preliminary culture of rectal contents, skin, and any septic lesions; careful sterilization of the skin with stringent asepsis and isolation of the rectum by a perineal wool pad; and prophylactic administration of penicillin to prevent gas gangrene, formerly a dreaded complication of leg amputations. The bowel should be emptied before operation. Frequent washing of the wound with saline during the operation and local antibiotics applied at the conclusion of the procedure are both measures which can reduce the incidence of local sepsis.

The operation recommended as most suitable at below-knee level is the long posterior flap amputation as first described by Kendrick (1956), combined with a myoplastic technique described by Burgess (1969). Recently we have changed to skew sagittal skin flaps combined with the myoplasty to produce a pre-shaped stump that allows early casting. During operation a minimum of diathermy is used and a minimum of foreign tissue buried. Skin hooks are used in preference to tissue forceps and absolute haemostasis must be secured. If there is any likelihood of a haematoma, suction drainage by fine plastic tube is recommended. Recently we have found that Steristrips are preferable to skin sutures. A light dry dressing can be applied and covered by a non-constricting 10 cm (4 in) crêpe bandage or light plaster. Any proximal constriction acts as a venous tourniquet and the resulting oedema may disrupt the tissues and be the precursor of infection. It is impossible to apply the traditional stump bandage without producing proximal constriction. The risk of sepsis in the ischaemic stump is greatest when the first dressing is changed and cross-infection may occur when the sutures are removed. These procedures should therefore be carried out in a sterile room or operating theatre whenever possible.

In some cases inevitably below-knee amputation is not possible and a through-knee amputation can be used with equal lateral flaps. These appear to have advantage over the traditional long anterior flap. Good results have been reported with the through-knee amputation in ischaemic disease. However, our own operative experience gives a 50% incidence of re-amputation for failed healing unless lateral skin flaps are utilized, when satisfactory results can be achieved.

The Gritti–Stokes and supracondylar amputation have excellent records for low mortality and primary wound healing. However, problems with subsequent non-union of the patella in Gritti–Stokes amputation, and prosthetic problems in both the supracondylar and Gritti–Stokes amputation, make us reluctant to use them. The stump in each case is narrow in cross-section. It cannot therefore restrain rotation of the prosthesis and although some end-bearing is feasible, the distal loading is very high and all or most of the body weight must be taken on the ischial tuberosity. This entails the use of a full-length prosthesis with an ischial seating of quadrilateral section, that is a similar prosthesis to that used for above-knee amputations and which elderly patients find so difficult to manage. Lastly, the knee-joint mechanism must be of an unsophisticated type constructed around the stump end, unless a four-bar linkage is incorporated.

Prostheses can be made and patients can walk with them after a supracondylar or Gritti–Stokes amputation, but our belief is that a below-knee amputation, when it can be done, makes the patient's life very much easier.

The ultimate decision on the level of amputation must be made according to the ability of the tissues to heal. Little help can be gained from the history or from clinical examination apart from observation of the level of pallor, coldness, and gangrene. The amputation must be through warm pink skin. Burger's test has no obvious correlation with the eventual level of amputation.

Much investigation has been made into ways of selecting the optimum level. Some correlation has been shown with the appearance on arteriography, and below-knee stumps are unlikely to heal if the profunda femoris is not patent. Studies with intra-arterial dyes give little more information than do the colour and temperature on clinical observation. Intra-arterial isotope injections and isotope clearance studies from the calf muscle have not proved to be of any significant assistance. Neither have skin thermometry or skin thermography; electromagnetic flow studies have been shown to indicate the likelihood of tissue healing. However, Yao and Irvine (1969) believe that systolic pressure in the ankle, measured by using an ultrasound detector over the posterior tibial artery and digital plethysmography, may prove to be the most accurate index of limb blood flow and this may well be correlated to the ability of a lower amputation to heal. An ankle systolic pressure less than 40 mmHg (5.5 kPa) makes it unlikely that a below-knee level of amputation will heal. Xenon clearance from an intradermal injection 10 cm below the tibial tubercle is a good guide to the ability of the tissues to heal at the below-knee level. Xenon clearance has problems with isotope storage and calibration. Amidopyrine clearance has given similar information but other methods are simpler in practical use. Skin diffusion oxymmetry is emerging as a reliable index of skin perfusion. The oxygen content of the healing skin is a limiting factor in the ability of an amputation stump to heal and the partial pressure of oxygen in the skin is critical. A value of less than 40 mmHg is usually incompatible with wound healing at that level.

In clinical practice at the present time, the colour and temperature of the skin before operation and the appearance of free capillary bleeding from the cut surfaces of the tissue at operation remain the best guide. It is therefore our practice to make the final decision of the level of amputation on the operating table.

Postoperative pain is an indication that the healing process is impaired by anoxia and likely to fail. Most patients comment that the pain of a recent amputation is much less than the original rest pain and this is an index of correct amputation level and technique.

If a healing stump is painful and healing delayed due to the selection of the incorrect level, there is no alternative to reamputation. Hyperbaric oxygen only delays the unpleasant decision and arterial procedures should already have given their maximum benefit.

Once healing of the amputation is obtained and rehabilitation is completed, the conditions of life for the patient must be controlled and all necessary help obtained from social services. The aim is to restore the patient to his own environment and to rehabilitate him to be active and, if possible, independent.

Meanwhile it must not be forgotten that the disease process which caused the amputation must be treated. Estimation of cholesterol, lipoproteins and triglyceride levels in the blood may indicate the need for dietary changes or specific therapy with cholestyramine or clofibrate. Polycythaemia and fibrinogen excess must be recognized and treated.

The deleterious effect of smoking is well recognized in thrombo-angiitis obliterans. Of patients with arteriosclerosis,

92% of all male amputees smoke but a much smaller number of female amputees are found to be smokers; however there is sufficient evidence to recommend the patient to stop smoking in an effort to slow the progress of any obliterative arterial disease.

Nevertheless, atheroma of sufficient severity to cause peripheral tissue loss is severe enough to be associated with other vascular catastrophes. A patient with an amputation and a cerebrovascular occlusion or a major coronary occlusion, if over the age of 60, is unlikely to survive for more than a year. Some evidence is emerging that the activity involved in walking with a prosthesis may improve the prognosis in these patients.

Occlusion of the deep veins of the leg or loss of valves and muscle function are not yet remediable by surgery. A proximal obstruction in the iliac veins or incompetent perforating veins along the leg can be treated by bypass or ligation respectively but otherwise the control of venous hypertension can only be palliative. Where a painful ulcer does not respond to elastic support, elimination of infection, and skin-graft cover, a below-knee amputation may provide renewed mobility, elimination of pain and improvement in general health. The main obstacle to this very effective treatment is the patient's acceptance of such a major procedure.

8

Amputation in Trauma and for Other Causes

It is clearly not possible to be specific about the desirability of amputation in any particular pathological state as there are so many other factors to be considered. The age and occupation of the patient, his general physical state, social circumstances and habitat, the availability of prosthetic services and a host of others may all influence the final decision. Nevertheless some broad guidelines can be laid down.

In malignant disease and in vascular disease amputation may be the only means of saving life. In general orthopaedic disorders, however, this is seldom the case and the essential

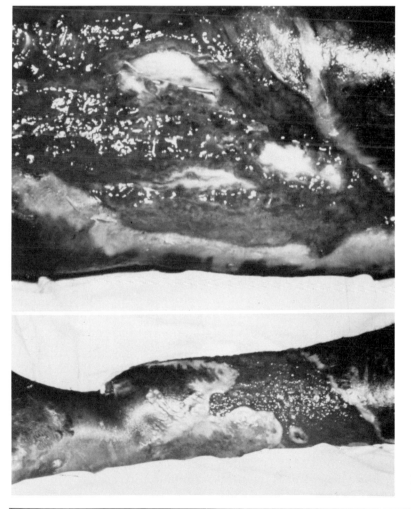

Fig. 8.1 Chronic osteomyelitis and non-union of tibial fractures following trauma

question is often whether or not the proposed prosthetic limb is more or less functional and aesthetically pleasing than the limb for which amputation is proposed.

The argument for and against amputation differs greatly in the upper and lower limbs. In the lower limb the ability to stand and at least walk are functions that most amputees can accomplish. In the upper limb the loss of the special qualities of grasp and prehension, but above all of sensation, is a serious disability; the replacement by a prosthesis, whilst conferring some relatively primitive movements such as pinching, gripping, pushing and pulling, cannot replace the upper limb as a sensory and tactile organ. It is for this reason above all others that amputation for functional reasons should seldom be performed in the upper limb. The loss of both arms forces the patient to use a prosthesis. The loss of one still leaves the patient with a choice. Despite the opinion of a number of limb-fitting surgeons that use is generally made of an upper-limb prosthesis, recent studies have shown that disappointingly few single-arm amputees use their prostheses regularly for work or daily living. Upper-limb prostheses are also disappointing cosmetically and whilst dress arms are often worn it is doubtful whether they are aesthetically preferable to a roughly normal, though functionless, arm.

If one is to lay down general rules, the upper limb should be preserved if it is not a danger to life and if it is not excruciatingly painful. There may be indications for amputation of an upper limb which is totally paralysed and anaesthetic, as in some brachial plexus injuries, but even here we believe that the present enthusiasm for this procedure should be tempered with considerable doubt. The much closer proximity of functional loss with the lower-limb ablation and its functional prosthetic replacement is such that amputation may be advised less hesitantly in a wide range of orthopaedic conditions.

INFECTIVE CONDITIONS

Acute

Amputation was at one time commonly performed as a life-saving measure in acute osteomyelitis but the efficacy of antibiotics and local limited surgery is such that this is seldom required today. Infection with the organisms causing gas gangrene was often rapidly fatal in the past and radical emergency amputation was the only means of saving life. The advent of antibiotics, particularly intracavity slow-release agents and, in some centres, the additional help of hyperbaric oxygen, has radically changed the picture. Whilst local and sometimes radical surgery are required, amputation is seldom necessary. In limbs which are basically ischaemic, however, amputation may still be mandatory.

Fig. 8.2 Gross deformity following chronic osteomyelitis

Chronic

Chronic osteomyelitis, affecting particularly the long bones such as the tibia and femur, is still commonly seen and despite continued medical and surgical efforts some cases fail to heal. Persistent offensive discharge, often associated with pain and episodes of subacute flare-ups, may be sufficiently disabling to justify amputation. Clearly if the infection is associated with other severe abnormalities, such as severe joint stiffness or loss of sensation in the foot, then the decision to amputate is easier and the functional loss is less. Rarely tuberculous infections of bone, usually complicated by infection with secondary organisms, are seen and amputation may be the only means of cure. Although this problem is now rare in Western society it is still one of the commonest surgical problems in many developing countries. Amyloid disease occurs as a result of long-standing persistent infection and may eventually prove fatal if the infective source is not removed. This is an additional factor in favour of amputation.

Leprosy

Leprosy is now eminently treatable but a number of cases still present with the neurological sequelae of perforating ulcers in the feet and chronic osteomyelitis. Local surgery may effect a cure but recurrent breakdowns are not uncommon and amputation may be necessary.

NEUROLOGICAL CONDITIONS

Poliomyelitis

Occasionally amputation is desirable. However, most patients with severe paralysis affecting, let us say, one leg cope adequately with a surgical boot and calliper. Whilst these may be heavy and cumbersome the patient has often worn them since childhood and is used to them. Generally with paralysis of this degree there is severe muscular weakness around the hip as well, particularly extensors and abductors, and, should an amputation be performed, control of the prosthesis is likely to be poor. The gait is likely to be awkward and cumbersome. A rigid pelvic band at least will probably be necessary to suspend the prosthesis so that the patient is unlikely to gain much in terms of comfort, function or cosmesis. A stronger case for amputation can be made in those relatively rare cases where the paralysis is more limited, for instance below the knee. The calf and foot are withered and useless, the limb may be short, necessitating a high boot, a fixed deformity in a bad position may be present, and the winter is dreaded because of painful and sometimes ulcerated chilblains. The loss of such a limb may indeed be welcomed by the patient and here there is likely to be considerable gain in terms of symptomatic relief, performance and cosmesis.

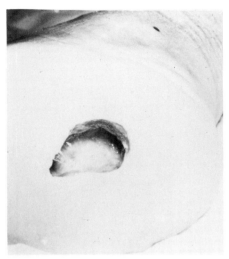

Fig. 8.3 Trophic ulceration in an anaesthetic foot associated with spina bifida

Other neurological conditions

These basic considerations apply to other paralytic states in the lower limb. If the paralysis is widespread and severe, as in some spinal injuries or in extensive myelomeningoceles, the ability to control a prosthesis is limited and only some other factor such as trophic ulceration would favour amputation. In this context amputation occasionally has a part to play in severe late stages of disseminated sclerosis. A useless limb, often with uncontrollable spasms and associated with severe contractures and gross ulceration around the trochanter and buttock, may be best treated by disarticulation at the hip joint rather than by local surgery. This has occasionally been performed and a long anterior flap extending almost to the knee consisting of much of the extensor mechanism and femoral artery and vein has been used to cover severe sacral sores which could not be closed by any other means.

Local neurological lesions such as division of the sciatic nerve can generally be controlled by a calliper and, provided that there is no gross fixed deformity of the foot, ulceration seldom occurs. A fixed deformity and ulceration would, however, favour amputation.

Many more cases of myelomeningocele now survive due to the combination of early closure of their spinal defect, Spitz–Holter valves for their hydrocephalus, and careful management of the urinary tract.

Whilst the primary orthopaedic aim must be directed to the preservation of limbs and the eradication of deformity by instrumental and surgical means, severe fixed or relapsing deformity possibly associated with ulceration and paralysis, particularly in the foot and ankle, may best be treated by amputation. As with other neurological conditions, however, considerable thought must be given to whether or not there will be skin with protective sensation on the stump or area of limb supporting the prosthesis. Also, because of frequent loss of hip extension and abduction, too much should not be hoped for in elegance of gait. Occasionally severe growth disturbance in this condition, associated with marked shortening of the limb, is a good indication for ablation.

Neurological conditions affecting particularly the sensory columns of the spinal cord, such as tertiary syphilis, present difficulties. Whilst the common peripheral manifestations of grossly unstable joints, particularly the knee and ankle often associated with ulcers, would seem ideal for amputation, the number of patients so treated who achieve satisfactory limb-wearing is small. Persistent problems with stump breakdown and severe disturbance of proprioception and other types of sensation too often commit the patient to a chairbound existence.

VASCULAR CONDITIONS

The main cause of amputation is atherosclerosis and this has been dealt with in Chapter 7. Two relatively uncommon vascular problems which do occasionally end in amputation are varicose ulceration and arteriovenous aneurysms. Severe persistent venous ulceration in the calf, which has persisted despite adequate treatment, may occasionally be sufficiently disabling and unpleasant to justify amputation. Gross arteriovenous manifestations are rarely seen affecting the limbs but the effect of these arteriovenous shunts may be so severe as to necessitate amputation. They may produce marked overgrowth of the limb, associated sometimes with fixed deformity (Klippel–Trenaunay syndrome). Persistent ulceration may eventually complicate the picture, and lurking in the background are the more general cardiovascular effects leading finally to a high-output heart failure.

It should be noted that, if the shunt is proximal in the thigh, this may preclude the wearing of a prosthesis.

MECHANICAL CONDITIONS

Arthritis

It is rare that arthritis in any form cannot be sufficiently controlled or relieved by conventional means but very occasionally ablation may be indicated for gross arthritic changes around the ankle and foot, particularly when surgery such as arthrodesis has failed to relieve pain, possibly because of failure of fusion. It is, however, in such conditions where pain is the sole symptom that the greatest care must be taken in advising amputation. The decision must be slow and deliberate and the patient must be fully aware of the limitations and problems associated with amputation. Seldom, if ever, should an amputation be performed without the patient having the opportunity to see and talk to several amputees with the same level of loss. Not only, as it were, should the patient take a second look but often the surgeon also should seek a second opinion. Such caution may seem unnecessary but a large number of amputees who suffer 'painful phantoms and painful stumps', and thus fail to be rehabilitated fully and also fail to become habitual limb-users, have had amputations for painful arthritic conditions, often secondary to trauma. Their inability to adapt to life as an amputee and the bitterness with which they regret having subjected themselves to the operation are intimately and often permanently entangled. Occasionally in severe arthritis in which both pain and instability are a problem, particularly where the instability is so severe that a neuropathic joint is suspected but unproven, and where adequate control cannot be obtained with callipers, amputation may be desirable, but these circumstances are very rare.

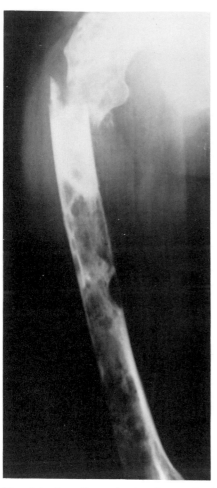

Fig. 8.4 A radiograph showing multiple pathological fractures due to metastases from carcinoma of the breast

Congenital deformities

Severe congenital deformities are a complex subject dealt with in chapter 16. Occasionally marked fixed congenital deformities, such as those seen in arthrogryphosis, may be helped by amputation but it is rare that the deformities are so severe that they cannot be corrected by other surgical means; then even if they are of only limited use since sensation is intact, they are preferable to prostheses. Neurofibromatosis, occasionally associated with pseudoarthrosis of the tibia, which usually fails to join despite repeated surgical attacks and in which the leg often becomes 10–15 cm (4–6 in) short, may best be treated by below-knee amputation.

Pathological fractures

Pathological fractures resulting from primary malignant tumours require amputation, but if they are due to non-malignant lesions of bone union can generally be obtained by conventional means. Pathological fractures through secondary deposits such as metastatic carcinoma of the breast can usually be stabilized and rendered painless by internal fixation with metal, assisted, if necessary, by acrylic cement. Amputation is best avoided because of the limited life expectation and the psychological trauma of amputation superimposed on a patient who is already dying. Uncontrollable pain from metastases may only be successfully treated by amputation and in these circumstances ablation is a welcome relief for the patient.

TRAUMATIC CONDITIONS

For convenience one may consider the question of amputation in trauma in three fundamental phases which may be called early, intermediate, and late.

Early amputation

This is required when the degree of destruction is so gross that there is no alternative to amputation. Situations where the limb is ischaemic, where there is considerable destruction or actual loss of its skin, bone and muscles, and where its nerve supply is severed do not leave any room for doubt and an amputation should be performed at the first opportunity. The wounds should be treated according to general surgical principles: vigorously and thoroughly cleaned with excision of all dead tissue but being particularly thorough with removal of dead muscle, fat and fascia, preserving however as much viable skin as possible. Dead bone must clearly be removed but as much viable bone as possible should be preserved initially, providing it looks practicable at some stage to cover it with skin. So much destruction, associated almost inevitably with serious wound contamination, precludes wound closure, which if practised will almost certainly result in serious infection and further tissue loss. The wound should be covered with a non-adherent dressing and considerable quantity of fluffed-up gauze. There is often a danger of skin retraction and if this is going to make delayed wound closure difficult then it must be kept to a minimum by two or three sutures covered with rubber tubes and tied over the dressings. The wound under these conditions heals safely and quickly. Further minor excision of sloughs may be required after three to four days, but often after about five days delayed primary suture can be undertaken. No attempt should be made to produce a formal myoplasty; skin cover is all that can be hoped for at this stage. Any areas that cannot be covered by skin closure should be grafted with split skin. Care must be taken that the donor skin sites are not those which may be in contact with a prosthesis. This is the quickest method of securing complete wound healing; by preserving the maximum length of stump it keeps the maximum surgical options open to the patient. Should the stump prove unsatisfactory in its shape, length or quality of skin cover, then a definitive operation at a minimally higher level can be performed. Any length of stump below the knee joint is worth preserving initially. The paper-thin unstable scars that may have resulted from split-skin grafting can readily be replaced by a cross-leg flap or tube pedicle, leaving the patient with his own functioning knee — a situation infinitely preferable to amputation at a higher level.

These considerations have been directed to injuries of the calf but the principles apply to other injuries of the lower limb and

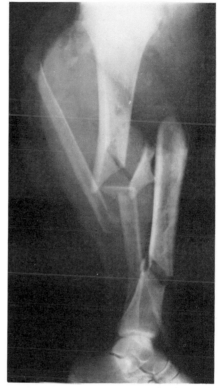

Fig. 8.5 A radiograph showing severe crush injury of the leg with vascular and neurological damage

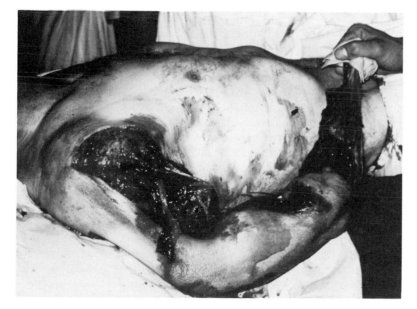

Fig. 8.6 Traumatic amputation of the arm with confused multiple wounds unsuitable for reimplantation

Fig. 8.7 Multiple injuries following a mine explosion

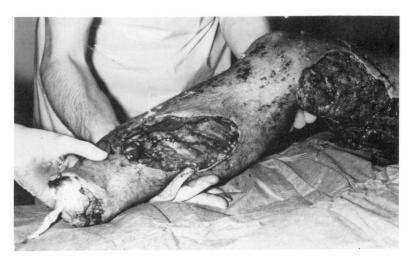

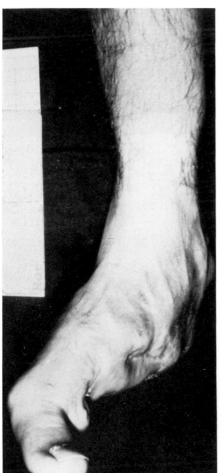

Fig. 8.8 Severe residual deformity after a road-traffic accident

upper limb as well. In the upper limb, the preservation of all possible length is most important and in particular all viable skin with intact sensation must be retained. This applies particularly in the hand and at the wrist where even the preservation of some crude stumpy remnant, providing it is covered with skin and has an intact sensation, may be put to some important use later by the patient. It may be preferable to a prosthesis and, used in conjunction with a simple post attached to a rigid bracelet on the forearm, more functional than a wrist disarticulation and a formal upper-limb prosthesis.

Intermediate amputation

The decision to amputate after ineffective attempts have been made to save the limb is often very difficult. Sometimes the issue becomes fairly clear. With clearly non-viable tissue, such as gangrenous toes, the inevitability of at least limited amputation soon becomes apparent to both surgeon and patient. Where the combination of injuries is gross, with perhaps extensive skin loss, wound infection, and gross bony and articular damage, the balance between prolonged surgical efforts with a dubious end result and limited recovery or early amputation and rapid rehabilitation presents a terrible choice, which is more often the doctor's than the patient's. In the upper limb almost any attempt at preservation is worth while but in the lower limb, particularly if the damage is restricted to below the knee and sensation is lost or severely impaired, then amputation should be more readily contemplated as an alternative solution. Experience is vital and second opinions often immensely helpful. A plea must be made for taking the decision reasonably early. Nothing is more disappointing for the patient than months of time wasted with numerous operations, internal fixation, sequestrectomies, cross-leg flaps, etc., and then the eventual choice of amputation. With so much time and suffering lost the difficulty of the decision for the patient is often that much greater.

Late amputation

The indications have largely been discussed earlier in relation to orthopaedics. Non-union may resist all surgical efforts, at least in the tibia, though very rarely in the femur. Pain and instability may be sufficiently disabling to justify amputation, although it is surprising how good function can be with an ununited tibia. Similarly, malunion is compatible with surprisingly good function and amputation is generally inadvisable.

Regrettably, the symptoms from these conditions are coloured by the background of legal compensation that lies behind many of these cases. When it is possible, it is generally better to have all claims settled before deciding whether or not symptoms justify amputation. A satisfactory medicolegal outcome sometimes has a remarkable ameliorating effect on symptoms.

9

Amputation in Neoplastic Disease

The decision to amputate a limb for neoplastic disease is always a distressing one as the patient is apparently healthy and the procedure inflicts an obvious disability. The indications for amputation in patients with tumours should therefore be considered carefully, whether the objective is surgical care or palliation of symptoms, and the right decision can only be made with a knowledge of the natural history of each neoplasm.

BENIGN TUMOURS

An amputation is occasionally required when the size or position of a benign tumour causes gross disorganization of function or intractable pain. Very large chondromas and neurofibromas can produce this situation, with involvement of the sciatic or brachial plexus. Local excision would leave a flail extremity and, particularly in the lower limb, amputation would be necessary. However, in the upper limb any function which remains after an extensive local excision may be of value. Every means of preserving partial function should be considered before amputation is selected; this implies full consultation between the surgeon, pathologist, prosthetist and orthopaedic surgeon to ensure that every procedure of orthotics, tendon transplantation and joint fixation is considered. The introduction of satisfactory bone prostheses has limited the occasions on which amputation will be needed. Recent developments in the field of orthotics have produced the light-weight 'S' forearm splint and motorized splints are being used experimentally.

MALIGNANT TUMOURS

These may be primary within the limb or secondary to tumour in other parts of the body; numerically, secondary metastases are the most frequent tumours to involve the limbs but amputation is only very rarely employed in their treatment.

Metastatic tumours

Metastases to the soft tissues and skin of a limb are rare unless there is widespread dissemination of the disease throughout the body and amputation would not be indicated in the terminal phase of the condition. However, in isolated cases a large metastasis causing pain might be an indication for palliative amputation if other methods of control had failed.

Where there is painful lymphoedema from node involvement removal will contribute to adequate palliation.

Where the primary tumour has been treated and controlled an isolated metastasis may be treated by excision; this situation occurs in renal carcinoma but may also apply in bowel adenocarcinoma.

Many metastatic tumours occur in the bones of the limbs, notably those of breast, prostate, lung, thyroid, kidney and adrenal cortex. Isolated renal carcinoma metastases are the only tumours in which amputation would be considered if an incomplete result followed radiotherapy but wherever possible local excision would be preferred. Fortunately the remainder are likely to respond to radiotherapy or cytotoxic agents. Those from breast, prostate and thyroid may respond to hormonal agents or hormonal ablation. Even a pathological fracture is better treated by internal fixation and radiotherapy than by amputation.

Primary tumours

Neoplasms which arise within the tissue of a limb require radical treatment; if there are no distant metastases the aim should be cure and long-term survival without compromise from functional considerations. This does not imply that amputation for malignant disease is the only surgery that is radical, nor does it mean that the surgical principles of a good amputation should be disregarded.

The diversity of behaviour of different types of limb tumour makes any generalization unsafe and it is necessary to consider the common types of primary malignant tumour which occur in the limbs.

Skin tumours

Malignant melanoma.
This skin tumour is frequently found on the legs and less often on the arms; benign pigmented moles on the sole of the foot and under the nails are liable to undergo malignant change. As malignant melanoma spreads through the subcutaneous lymphatics to the regional lymph nodes and to the skin around the primary site to form satellite nodules, radical clearance necessitates removal of a wide area of skin and subcutaneous tissue; only in the digits is amputation needed. Malignant melanoma has a sinister reputation but cures can be obtained by adequate and careful early treatment and the prognosis can be predicted by the grading of tumour thickness and cell pattern, although blood-borne metastases may appear at any time during the course of the disease.

Biopsy should be performed if there is any doubt concerning the diagnosis but it should be avoided if possible. Biopsy should take the form of complete excision with a clearance of 5 mm of normal tissue; this must not be performed under local anaesthetic as this will risk implantation of tumour cells. Frozen section may be satisfactory but it is often necessary to wait for a paraffin-embedded section, in which case the wound is closed with small sutures.

Primary excision of a malignant melanoma should remove the lesion in an ellipse of skin and subcutaneous fat and fascia, to clear the melanoma by at least 5 cm (2 in) laterally and below, and by 15 cm (6 in) in the line of the lymphatic drainage. This leaves a wide defect which must be covered by a partial-thickness skin graft. Where the melanoma lies close to the regional lymph-node group a block dissection is performed in continuity with the primary excision. Routine prophylactic block dissection has been replaced by the administration of intralymphatic iodine-131 Lipiodol, but where there are enlarged regional lymph nodes a block dissection should be performed to clear them.

Inoculation of smallpox vaccine into tumour nodules has had some limited success and immunotherapy can produce occasional remission, but the best control of subcutaneous dissemination in the limb has been obtained with isolated limb perfusion using a pump oxygenator and this has had a considerable role in avoiding amputation. Radiotherapy has a place in the control of malignant melanoma and cytotoxic chemotherapy continues to increase in efficacy.

These principles apply to a malignant melanoma of a digit but amputation gives better clearance and function afterwards. The whole digit and metatarsal or metacarpal must be cleared, together with an area of skin from the dorsum of the foot or hand in which the lymphatics run. This area will require partial-thickness skin grafting.

A particular problem is the subungual melanoma, which may cause difficulties in diagnosis; a few days' observation should distinguish it from a subungual haematoma, and nothing less than amputation of the digit is adequate for the treatment. Malignant melanoma of the sole of the foot can be well treated by wide excision and partial-thickness grafting, as already described. Split skin can make an adequate covering for the sole.

On rare occasions when there is extensive uncontrolled malignant melanoma of a limb, recurrent nodules along the lymphatic channels, uncontrolled tumour at the primary site and regional nodes involved, some fungating through the skin causing pain and distress, a palliative amputation may relieve the symptoms. Careful judgement is required as the disease may recur in the stump before pulmonary metastases appear, and if pulmonary metastases are already present medication may provide better palliation.

Epithelioma.
Squamous carcinoma arising as a spontaneous lesion is highly radiosensitive and amenable to radiotherapy or surgical excision. However, the squamous carcinoma arising in a venous ulcer,

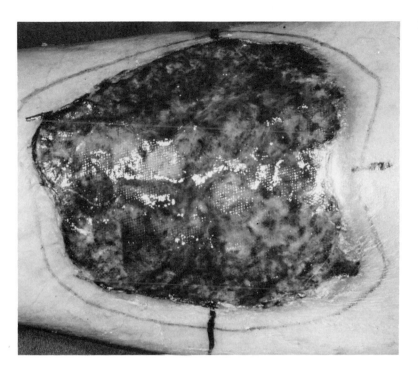

Fig. 9.1 Marjolin's ulcer

osteomyelitic sinus or burn scar (Marjolin's ulcer) (Fig. 9.1) can behave in a very aggressive manner and should be treated by biopsy and radiotherapy; unless response is complete, amputation well clear of the ulcer and above the bone underlying the tumour is required. Where the regional lymph nodes are invaded these should be treated by block dissection or radiotherapy, according to the state of the patient.

Actinic cancers of the hands and occupational cancers of the hand in those who work with radioactive materials and X-rays pose special problems and wide areas of skin may be affected by premalignant changes. Therefore excision and partial-thickness grafting of wide areas is preferable to amputation, but where invasion or destruction of phalanges has occurred amputation of digits may be necessary. Excision is preferred to irradiation in skin already unstable, but in extreme old age or intercurrent disease this risk may be accepted.

Basal cell carcinoma.
Rodent ulcers of the limbs are very rare and can be readily treated by wide excision; one case occurring on the nail bed required amputation of the distal phalanges of the digit. Rodent ulcers are radiosensitive and can be treated by biopsy and superficial irradiation. Lymphatic spread is not a characteristic of this tumour.

Intra-epidermal carcinoma (Bowen's disease).
This slowly progressive condition can occur on the limbs and can

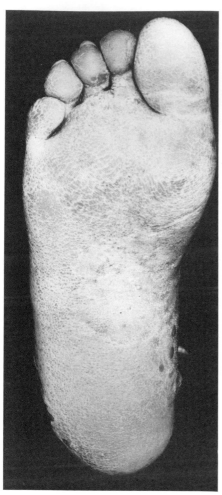

Fig. 9.2 Kaposi's sarcoma

always be treated by excision and partial-thickness skin grafting to the defect.

Kaposi's sarcoma (see Fig. 9.2).
This tumour is rare in races other than the African Bantu; haemorrhagic nodules develop in the skin of the foot and lower limb, progressing to lymphoedema, lymph node involvement and distant metastases. The condition was formerly treated by amputation, but much better results are now being obtained with chemotherapy and irradiation.

Dermatofibrosarcoma protruberans.
In this sarcoma of the fibrous tissue of the dermis raised nodules and nodular infiltration of the skin may be discrete or over a wide area. The limbs are not often involved and wide excision and grafting eliminates the need for amputation.

Soft tissue tumours
Soft tissue sarcomas are not common but they occur frequently in the limbs, usually in patients under the age of 50. The histological appearances are difficult to interpret and the nomenclature is complex; the degree of malignancy is often underestimated and recurrence after inadequate treatment is all too frequent.

In general, soft tissue sarcomas metastasize by the bloodstream and spread by local invasion along tissue planes, especially along the muscle sheaths. Lymphatic involvement is an infrequent feature of these tumours. The encapsulated appearance of some tumours can be misleading and the tumour may have spread widely beyond these borders.

The high incidence of local recurrence might suggest that amputation should be performed more often, but adequate surgery short of amputation can produce good results. Accurate diagnosis by biopsy is essential and this is best obtained by deep incision with removal of an adequate piece of tumour. The skin incision should be small to minimize the chance of later fungation through the scar.

A further safeguard is to give pre-biopsy radiotherapy; 1000 rad in a single dose on the day of biopsy is cytostatic without effect on the histology and time can then be allowed for the processing of a paraffin section. The operative procedure should be carefully planned and the tumour fully assessed by radiography, including ultrasound examination, angiography and chest radiographs; examination at the time of biopsy under general anaesthetic is particularly valuable.

Wide surgical excision is required, with inclusion of the biopsy scar and the whole length of the muscle group with which the tumour is associated. This frequently constitutes a compartmental clearance, e.g. the posterior compartment of the lower leg for a fibrosarcoma of the soleus, which includes the gastrocnemius to its attachment to the femur. Frozen section specimens from the periphery of the excision should be examined as an additional

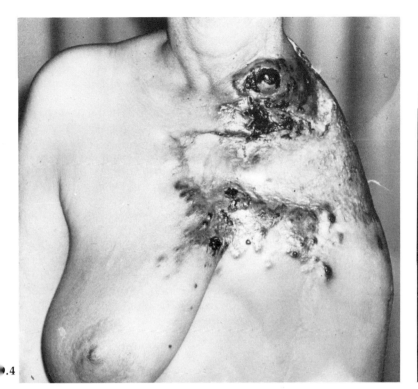

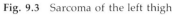

Fig. 9.3   Sarcoma of the left thigh
Fig. 9.4   Recurrence of a sarcoma in the amputation area
Fig. 9.5   Fibrosarcoma of the right hip before and after amputation

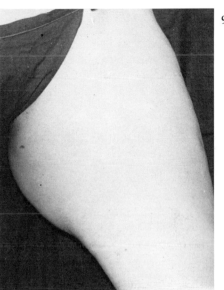

9.3

9.4

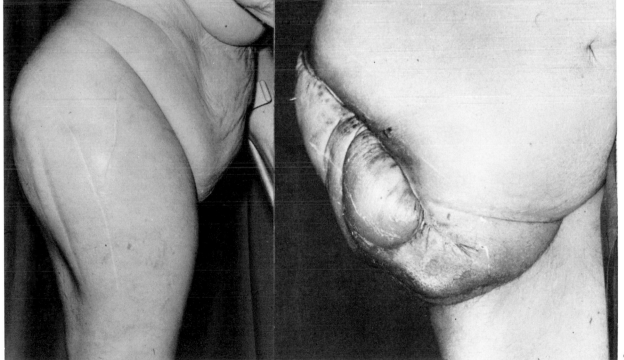

9.5

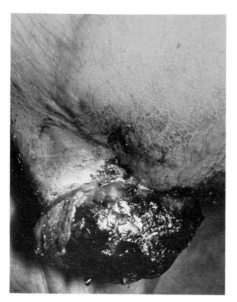

Fig. 9.6   Recurrence of fibrosarcoma at the site of amputation

safeguard. Only when such an excision would produce a useless extremity is amputation required, e.g. a synoviosarcoma of the lower leg invading all the muscular compartments would require a through-knee amputation. Even when amputation is indicated, the same principle of clearance of the whole length of a muscle or bone must be observed.

The first treatment of soft tissue sarcoma offers the best chance of cure; therefore preoperative irradiation, biopsy followed by wide excision and occasionally amputation and postoperative irradiation should be the plan of treatment in most cases. In-adequate excision leads to local recurrence, often with progressive aggressiveness of the tumour and increasing chance of blood-borne pulmonary metastases.

Fibrosarcoma.
This varies from the solid white fibroma, which is rarely truly benign, to the anaplastic soft tumour, which grows rapidly, is extremely vascular and spreads early through the bloodstream to the lungs. The general principles which have been discussed apply and amputation is only required when clearance cannot otherwise be obtained. The aggressive fibromatoses are managed in the same way.

Liposarcoma and angiosarcoma.
Both occur rarely in the limbs but when they do so they infiltrate the tissues diffusely and wide excision is not often feasible; therefore amputation after radiotherapy is more often employed.

Lymphangiosarcoma.
This rare spontaneous tumour is seen most frequently after clearance of the axilla in radical mastectomy for mammary carcinoma. The arm is brawny due to invasion of axillary lymph nodes by mammary carcinoma, accompanied by axillary vein occlusion. The whole arm is grossly swollen and a forequarter amputation is necessary to obtain even palliation of symptoms.

Rhabdomyosarcoma.
This is usually a fast-growing tumour seen in young patients. It affects the limbs less often than the trunk. Wide invasion often prevents excision by compartmental clearance, and amputation and radiotherapy are required.

Neurofibrosarcoma.
This form generally occurs in a pre-existing neurofibroma, in particular in generalized neurofibromatosis (von Reckling-hausen's disease). Wide excision is required with a considerable length of the nerve, as extension along the nerve is the rule. If the tumour is very large or involves a nerve plexus then amputation may be the only method of treatment. Forequarter or hindquarter amputation is performed if brachial or sciatic plexuses are involved and the tumour mass can be cleared.

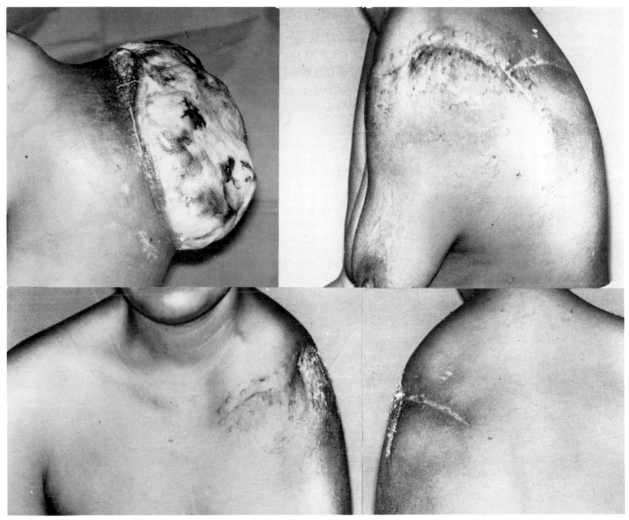

Synoviosarcoma.

Developing from joints and tendon sheaths, particularly in the fingers and hand, and also from the knee joint, this tumour may be found at any site in the limbs. A high proportion of these tumours are very active and in general the prognosis is not good, but the same principles of treatment apply. As many of these tumours involve the digits, amputation is necessary well clear of the mass.

Tumours of bone

Bone tumours constitute the most frequent indication for amputation in the treatment of malignant disease of the limbs. The frequency of metastatic bone tumours has been emphasized and therefore no amputation should be performed without an adequate biopsy.

Fig. 9.7   A forequarter amputation for fibro-sarcoma of the shoulder

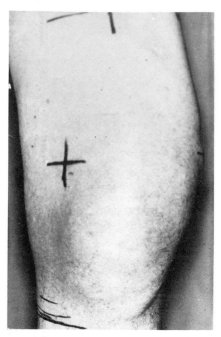

Fig. 9.8 Synoviosarcoma of the left knee

Osteosarcoma.

The most aggressive primary tumour of bone, this occurs in young patients unless it appears in the course of osteitis deformans (Paget's disease of bone). Originally defined as a malignant tumour of bone cells, it may be osteoblastic, chondroblastic or fibroblastic in type. Each of these must be distinguished from the corresponding differentiated sarcoma, which in every case has a better prognosis.

Osteosarcoma occurs, in order of greatest frequency, in the femur, tibia and humerus, but rarely in the pelvis and jaws. The majority of osteosarcomas therefore affect the lower limb, the lower end of the femur and the upper end of the tibia.

The rate of growth and early blood-borne dissemination to produce pulmonary metastases are the features which are responsible for the poor prognosis. The early appearance of pulmonary metastases marks the failure of local treatment to control the disease. Many of the metastases are developing at the time the patient presents for treatment; in these patients amputation adds distress to the short period of survival and it has therefore been the practice at Westminster Hospital, London, and at Queen Mary's Hospital, Roehampton, to select for amputation only those patients who do not have early metastases.

The programme of treatment instituted by Sir Stanford Cade consists of the primary treatment of the osteosarcoma by megavoltage (2 MV) radiotherapy, 7000 to 8000 rad in seven to eight weeks. Open incision biopsy is performed during the first week of treatment. This is done through a small incision with a tourniquet if it can be applied without any pressure on the tumour. Unfortunately the application of a tourniquet will not prevent blood-borne metastases at the time of operation as the free communication between the medullary cavity and the venous system cannot be controlled; a pertrochanteric venogram is convincing evidence of this fact. However, in tumours below the knee it may be of some value, but an Esmarch type should not be used as it would compress the tumour and cause dissemination. The patient is then observed until three or four months have elapsed from the commencement of treatment; if there is no radiological evidence of pulmonary metastases, amputation is carried out. The level of amputation must be such that there is no risk of local recurrence in the stump; therefore the whole bone which is involved must be removed. Transection of a bone invaded by osteosarcoma has been found to lead to recurrence in the cut end, thought to be due to intramedullary spread. This dictates hip disarticulation for osteosarcoma of the upper end of the femur, above-knee amputation for osteosarcoma of the upper end of the tibia, to clear the attachment of the gastrocnemius, and through-knee amputation for osteosarcoma of the lower end of the tibia. When the humerus is involved the shoulder is disarticulated unless invasion has occurred around the shoulder joint. Osteosarcoma of the forearm bones requires disarticulation at the elbow.

An alternative has been advocated by Platt, in which a very high dose of high-voltage radiotherapy is applied in excess of the tolerance of the normal tissues and this is followed immediately by amputation. If high-voltage radiotherapy is not available the only treatment can be immediate amputation, but the same considerations of level apply.

The published five-year survival rates vary between 5% and 35%. There are many factors which make comparisons dangerous but there does not appear to be any statistical disadvantage to patients if amputation is done some time after radiotherapy.

Osteogenic sarcoma.

In several trial studies chemotherapy has been shown to have a significant effect on primary bone tumours affecting the limbs. Although initial results only have been published it seems likely that intra-arterial chemotherapy with doxorubicin, combined with high-dose intermittent methotrexate administration and radiotherapy to the tumour, may exert sufficient control on tumour growth to render obsolete the previous concepts of amputation in selected patients who have no evidence of pulmonary metastases. It is likely that the management of these tumours will be a single cytostatic dose of radiotherapy performed hours before an adequate incision biopsy; following biopsy the patient will have intra-arterial doxorubicin combined with an effective course of radiotherapy. Then resection of affected bone, in the case of bone tumours, or soft tissue muscle group, in the case of soft tissue sarcomas, will allow graft or prosthetic reconstruction of the affected bone with limb preservation. Repeated doses of intra-arterial doxorubicin are administered and long-term chemotherapy is applied with oral methotrexate, given to a maximum dose. Folinic acid rescue may be necessary to prevent bone marrow inhibition. It is likely that the chemotherapy routine will be improved but the concept of limb preservation represents a major change in treatment policy and will leave only the largest tumours and those which fail to respond to be treated by amputation and prosthetic replacement.

Periosteal fibrosarcoma.

This tumour has many of the characteristics of an osteosarcoma, but the bone involvement is by invasion and this is a less aggressive tumour. Nevertheless full combined treatment by radiotherapy, biopsy and ablation of the whole bone is required. This usually entails an amputation, but chemotherapy may give the opportunity for limb salvage.

Ewing's tumour of bone.

This eponym probably covers reticulum cell tumour of bone and metastatic neuroblastoma. These produce a well-recognized radiological appearance with bone destruction and onion-peel subperiosteal bone formation. Biopsy is often inconclusive and every case should be fully investigated, including assessment of

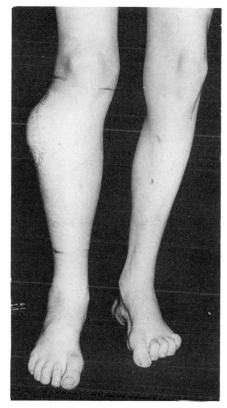

Fig. 9.9 Osteogenic sarcoma of the right fibula

urinary catecholamines, to exclude a neuroblastoma.

These tumours are highly radiosensitive and only the very occasional case which recurs or fails to respond would require amputation.

Chondrosarcoma (malignant enchondroma).

This tumour must be distinguished from chondroblastic osteosarcoma. It occurs later in life, 30 to 50 years, and affects the long bones, pelvis and ribs. Chondrosarcoma is slow growing and remains locally invasive for many years but ultimately dissemination causes pulmonary metastases. The tumours are minimally radiosensitive and should be treated by removal of the affected bone and adjacent soft tissues, in most cases involving amputation above the involved bone. Most hindquarter amputations are performed for this tumour.

Plasmacytoma (myeloma).

If solitary, this tumour is the precursor of a widespread disease, multiple myelomatosis, which may be regarded as a diffuse neoplasm of the immunologically active cells of the bone marrow, also producing abnormal proteins in the blood and urine. Amputation therefore has no place in the treatment. The local tumour is radiosensitive and the general disease can be controlled with cytotoxic drugs such as melphalan.

Osteoclastoma (giant cell tumour of bone).

This tumour is seen between the ages of 10 and 30; it occurs in the distal femur, proximal tibia, distal radius, proximal humerus, distal ulna and proximal fibula, but rarely in the vertebrae or pelvis. The soap bubble appearance of a tumour expanding the bone is characteristic on the X-ray. Histology shows obvious giant cells, but it is impossible to distinguish with accuracy between the benign and malignant osteoclastoma unless there is hyperparathyroidism. For this reason malignancy should be assumed and the affected portion of the bone excised and reconstructed by bone graft or prosthesis. The fibula can be excised without replacement. Rapid growth or early recurrence may be the only evidence of a malignant osteoclastoma; in this case amputation with preliminary radiation will give the best chance of cure. The role of chemotherapy has yet to be assessed.

Visceral cancer

Carcinoma of the bladder, the uterine cervix, and the rectum spread to the lymph nodes of the lateral pelvic wall and direct spread may result in sciatic nerve plexus involvement with intractable pain and often incontinence. These complications may appear before metastases have developed in lungs and liver, allowing the disease to be encompassed by resection of the pelvis. This procedure has been carried out and named hemicorporectomy or translumbar amputation. The trunk is transected at the level of the fourth lumbar vertebra and a long posterior flap closes the peritoneum below. Preliminary formation of an ileal conduit for urine and a terminal colostomy is required. Several patients have been rehabilitated to a wheelchair existence and remained free of disease. A specially formed seat is required to provide stability and avoid high pressure areas of contact. The indications for this procedure can only be assessed for each individual patient and it must be considered only in those patients who have more than usual fortitude and determination.

10

Upper Limb Amputations
and Prostheses

THE HAND

Almost all amputations in the hand result from trauma. Rarely does infection cause a contracture sufficient to justify amputation. Occasionally, contracture of the little finger associated with Dupuytren's contracture is best treated by amputation.

Amputations of the hand can be properly discussed only within the context of the management of hand injuries and this is beyond the scope of this book. Nevertheless it is appropriate to establish a few guidelines where some limited amputation has to be performed. Too often hand injuries are considered commensurate in importance with their size, often being dealt with in minor casualty departments by inexperienced staff. Mismanagement, however, may be disproportionately disabling, with prolonged treatment and difficult rehabilitation necessitating the loss of many months of work.

In general, as much viable tissue as possible should be preserved after hand injury and partial amputation. This view must, however, be tempered with an appreciation of what will remain functional. The retention of a finger or part of one which is anaesthetic, cold and stiff does no service to the patient; it will discourage active use of the hand and ability to work, even after amputation. Pain, coupled with a lack of desire to return to normal function, will persist.

Amputation of digits

Generally the level will be determined by the degree of injury. If the injury is solely to the index or little finger, useful function is unlikely unless one-and-a-half phalanges are still present. Even at this level initial acceptance of this limited loss by the patient is often transmuted into a desire for cosmesis and later an amputation is requested. The best cosmesis is achieved by amputation through the metacarpal shaft with suitable bevelling. This, however, reduces the span of the hand and power of the grip and so it may be better in largely manual workers to amputate through the metacarpophalangeal joint.

The long and ring fingers are best amputated through whatever level will leave a mobile and comfortable stump. Even a very short stump, for example the proximal phalanx, may have some definite functional value and in the half-closed position may be at least cosmetically acceptable. Amputations of either of these fingers in which the metacarpal ray is excised for cosmetic

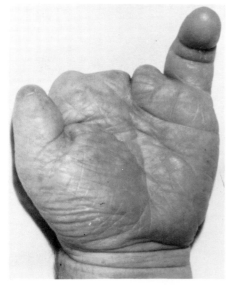

Fig. 10.1 Amputation of three digits and the distal phalanx of the thumb

reasons may seriously disturb function and are seldom desirable.

As much of the thumb as can be must be preserved for as long as possible. Any stump covered with sensitive skin may be of great value.

Technique. The level is generally determined by the trauma. The surgical objective is to produce a comfortable stump in which the end is covered with sensitive and supple skin.

The skin flaps must be of adequate length; if stretched and sutured tightly over the bone end, a painful and sensitive scar will be produced. Sufficient bone resection must be allowed. If possible the scar should be on the dorsum, which means using a slightly larger palmar flap. The extensor and flexor tendons should be allowed to retract: suturing these over the bone end will tether the flexor profundus and interfere with the function of the other fingers. Digital nerves should be pulled down, sectioned and allowed to retract away from the scar. The bone should be smoothed off, and in a disarticulation through an interphalangeal joint the condyles of the phalanx should be trimmed to reduce the bulk of the tip.

Multiple finger amputations, or injuries of such severity that several digits are injured, require skilled attention. Primary treatment must be directed to the preservation of as much tissue as possible. The final levels, types and number of amputations required will be determined by numerous factors such as the age and occupation of the patient, the possibility of reconstruction by skin grafting, neurovascular island flaps, pollicization of the index, etc., and the determination of the patient to achieve as good a result as possible.

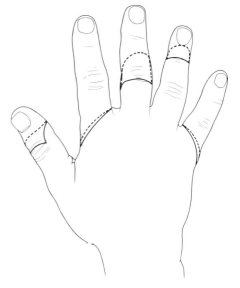

Fig. 10.2   Digital amputations. Incisions

Prostheses for mutilated hands

Single digit loss

It is usual for those who have lost part of a digit to want it artificially replaced early on in their adaptation to its loss. Special thimble-fitting digits can be, and are, supplied. They cannot be firmly attached to the digital stump and so provide no mechanical grip. They are bulkier than the normal digits because they have to fit over the stump and they cannot change colour to maintain the same appearance as the changing normal skin. The patient soon realizes that when others view the natural hand the flexed position of the fingers hides its terminal joints so that their presence or absence is not noticed, whereas the artificial digit is a physical encumbrance and an advertisement of the loss. Nevertheless, although a few continue to be used, the supply of a thimble-fitting digit may be therapeutic in enabling the patient to become reconciled to the loss.

Mutilated hands with residual digits

As with other levels of amputation it is usual to provide a

prosthesis which is either primarily cosmetic, for example a dress hand, or primarily functional, such as a working hand. The presence of residual digits presents some difficulties in preserving appearance: even if they are themselves unblemished they draw attention to the artificiality of the device and suitable openings have to be left in the prosthesis. Nevertheless any sensory mobile digit is of inestimable value as it provides sensation and grip. If the thumb is preserved and all the fingers are lost, then artificial ones can be fitted and the thumb may oppose against the index. If function rather than appearance is required a simple metal opposition plate with a serrated or pockled rubber face will afford a good grip. A splined nipple for attaching tools can be placed on the palmar surface if digital prehension is inadequate. Loss of the whole thumb, serious as it may seem, is best left untreated provided full mobility of the remaining fingers is maintained.

Mutilated hands with loss of all digits

Two versions of prostheses are supplied for these amputations. One is a cosmetic hand for dress purposes only. It has to contain the natural flesh and is therefore bulkier than the normal hand.

There are two types of functional prosthesis, the simplest being an opposition device consisting of a blocked leather wrist-strap incorporating a shaped metal plate faced either with pockled rubber or reversed chrome leather. The mobile palm remnant can then flex against it and hold light objects, thus preserving normal tactile sensibility. It has the merit that it preserves much of the available sensory area but does not give a sufficiently strong grip for wielding tools. The alternative is a strong blocked leather palm case with a castellated or screw nipple fitting into which the various tool attachments or a split hook can be fixed. A shoulder harness is necessary if a split hook or other body-activated appliance is to be used.

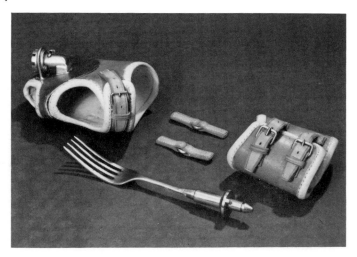

Fig. 10.3 A prosthesis for a partially mutilated hand, with wrist gauntlet and key snap fitting, and a table fork with adaptor

The attachments for these functional prostheses are numerous and depend on the bulbous nature of the stump and the use to which it will be put. When the metacarpals are retained the stump expands beyond the wrist and an opening in the palmar aspect of the socket facilitates this application. The opening can be closed by a press stud or strap and buckle. If the stump is not sufficiently bulbous to hold the appliance firmly the socket may be extended as a gauntlet to include the wrist joint and the lower quarter of the forearm, with the added disadvantage that it will then restrict wrist movement. For the latter to be retained additional suspension is sometimes afforded by the addition of an above-wrist band secured with side chapes to the main prosthesis.

A shoulder harness with an operating cord is necessary if an activated appliance such as a split hook is to be used. A purely cosmetic prosthesis usually takes the form of an appropriate glove filler with the necessary number of digits.

When all digits have been irreparably damaged serious consideration should be given to a disarticulation of the wrist since both function and cosmesis can more ably be restored.

Fig. 10.4 Amputation through the wrist. 1. The skin incision. 2. Structure encountered during disarticulation

THE WRIST

Disarticulation at the wrist

Indications for wrist disarticulation are rare but usually related to severe trauma to the hand with considerable loss of tissue and

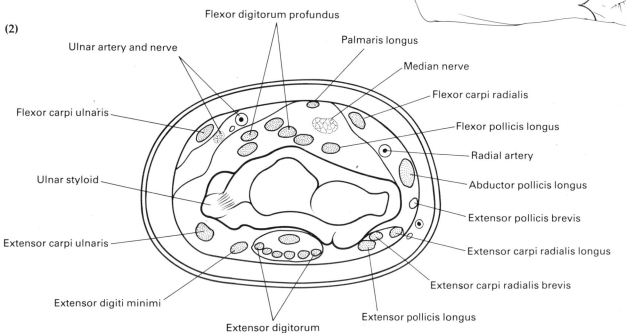

(1)

(2)

Flexor digitorum profundus

Ulnar artery and nerve

Palmaris longus

Median nerve

Flexor carpi ulnaris

Flexor carpi radialis

Flexor pollicis longus

Radial artery

Ulnar styloid

Abductor pollicis longus

Extensor pollicis brevis

Extensor carpi ulnaris

Extensor carpi radialis longus

Extensor carpi radialis brevis

Extensor digiti minimi

Extensor pollicis longus

Extensor digitorum

loss of all digits. Preserving any of the carpus will be a disadvantage for successful prosthetic replacement.

Technique. No special preoperative preparation is required. General anaesthesia is preferred and a tourniquet should be used.

The skin incision is commenced 1 cm (0.4 in) distal to the styloid processes. It is extended over the dorsal and palmar surfaces of the hand so that a long anterior flap of tough yet sensitive palmar skin is fashioned with a short dorsal flap. The flaps, together with the fascia, are reflected proximally to display the radiocarpal joint. The radial and ulnar arteries are divided and ligatured. The median, ulnar and radial nerves are drawn down and divided. The tendons are divided, leaving sufficient length so that opposing flexor and extensor muscles may later be sutured to each other. Soft tissue structures completing the radial carpal joint are divided.

The tourniquet is released and haemostasis secured. The amputation is finished by palpating the radial and ulnar styloids. If they are particularly prominent through the skin they should be carefully rounded off. Opposing flexor and extensor tendons are sutured to each other. This provides additional cover for the bone ends and, by providing isometric contraction for the muscle, helps to preserve the volume of the forearm. Fascia and skin are approximated by interrupted sutures. Suction drainage is used and wool and a light plaster shell are applied as dressings.

Prostheses for amputations at the wrist

Until recently amputation at wrist level was deplored by those working in the prosthetic field because it is impractical to use the standard adaptors and rotaries until the amputation is 5 cm above the wrist joint. A forearm socket utilizing the residual forearm rotation had not been devised. This is an example of the need for a surgeon to know the current prosthetic possibilities for his patient and his need to avoid complacency so that advances are made in prosthetics to meet what is otherwise good surgical practice.

Disarticulation at or near the wrist is now acceptable prosthetically, although all the problems are not yet satisfactorily solved. Improved methods of attaching artificial hands and appliances have made it easier to make use of this level and to interchange the appliances. As an amputation it has the great merit that it retains voluntary normal pronation and supination. Previously the sockets used almost or wholly obliterated this movement. Now split sockets are used which retain the forearm rotation. An accurate close-fitting socket of laminated plastic or blocked leather is made to a cast to enclose the distal 8–10 cm of the stump. A blocked leather cuff is made for the proximal 7–10 cm of the forearm. Two straps are then attached on either side between these two parts of the socket, holding the distal part on to the

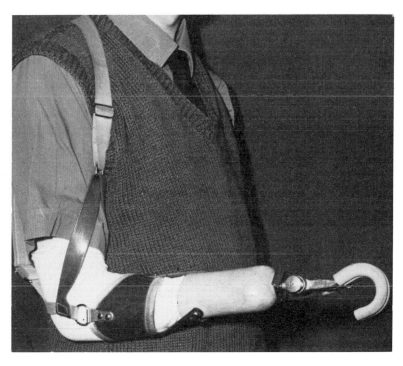

stump but allowing a full range of rotation. The normal suspension for a forearm prosthesis is then attached to the proximal cuff (see Fig. 10.5).

THE FOREARM

The usual indications for amputation through the forearm are for severe trauma affecting the wrist and hand and occasionally it is used as treatment for chronic sepsis or tumour of the hand.

Ideally, as with other amputations, the stump should be of reasonable length. A very long stump, whilst having the advantage of a long lever, often suffers from cold and cyanotic skin with little subcutaneous and muscular tissue covering the bone ends. The cosmesis is consequently poor; therefore the ideal length of stump is 17 cm, measured from the olecranon in the average adult, and this roughly corresponds to the junction of the proximal two-thirds and the distal one-third of the forearm.

Technique. No special preoperative preparation is required. General anaesthesia is preferred and a tourniquet is used.

The arm is held on the operating table in mid-supination. Skin flaps are fashioned from the extensor and flexor surfaces of the forearm commencing proximally at the proposed level of bone section. The deep fascia is raised with the skin flaps both anteriorly and posteriorly. The forearm muscles are sectioned 2–3 cm distal to the proposed line of bone section. The median, ulnar and radial nerves are gently pulled down and sectioned so that they

(1)

(2)

retract proximally into the forearm. Vessels are ligated and the radius and ulna divided with a saw, care being taken to round off the bone ends with a file.

The tourniquet is released and haemostasis is secured. The muscles are now sutured over the bone end at normal tension, the number of muscles sutured being determined by the bulk which must not be excessive. The fascia and skin are sutured in interrupted layers and the wound is drained with a suction drain.

The wound is dressed and the forearm encased in a padded light plaster of Paris cast. This is most comfortable and helps to control the stump volume. This technique may have to be slightly modified depending upon the level of section in the forearm.

Prostheses for forearm amputations

In the United Kingdom there has been a differentiation between long and short forearm stumps. If section is made at less than 5 cm proximal to the wrist joint there is a dual disadvantage. Pronation and supination have been lost and therefore the wrist disarticulation type of prosthesis which allows this movement is not suitable. Because of the length of the stump the conventional cosmetic hand cannot be used as it would hang lower than the natural limb. A rather short and stubby hand, therefore, has to be supplied and the wrist unit is visible below the cuff.

In practice, the level of the rotary in the long stump must be at wrist level. It may be at wrist level as a matter of choice in the shorter stump. The nearer the load is to the stump the shorter the lever on which it acts, producing less pressure on the end of the stump. The manual worker who takes off his coat and rolls up his sleeves will therefore want a bisection of the artificial forearm with the rotary as close to his stump as possible. But the clerical worker who wears a sleeved shirt and coat finds it an added disability to try to insert a change of appliance at mid-forearm; he will prefer to have a wrist bisection with some loss of appearance and mechanical disadvantage.

The use of a close-fitting inner cup socket gives more intimate contact between the stump and the prosthesis and is necessary for short stumps and longer ones which tend to be conical.

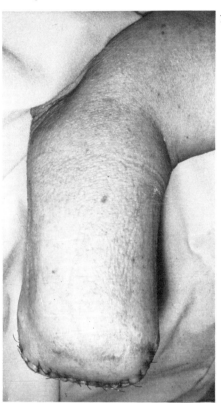

Fig. 10.7 A below-elbow myoplastic amputation stump
Fig. 10.8 Suspension straps for a below-elbow prostheses

10.7

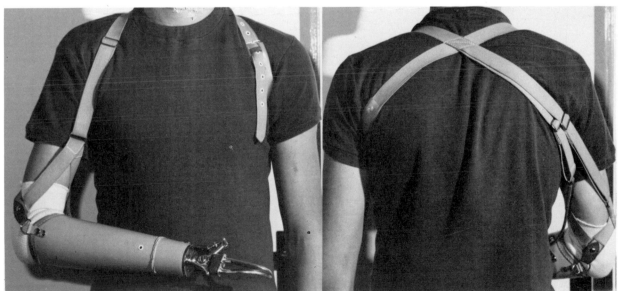

10.8

Sockets are made of either leather or plastic and the former is preferable for people engaged in hot and/or heavy manual work. The plastic, however, is to be preferred when lightness is a factor, particularly for people with very short stumps.

The below-elbow prosthesis can be self-suspending but if a mechanical hand, split hook or other activated appliance is to be used it is necessary to have some form of harness with an appropriate operating cord. Patients with weak triceps or biceps may need to be fitted with jointed side steels attached to a broad above-elbow corset. A locking device is incorporated to permit the elbow to be fixed in a variety of different positions thus permitting heavy lifting and activation of the terminal devices by means of a Bowden cable control.

If paralysis results in a flail shoulder then an arthrodesis should be considered provided the serratus anterior is fully active.

With normal shoulder musculature many below-elbow amputees can achieve a force varying from 10 to 30 kg when pulling on a cord which will open either a split hook or other activated terminal device. Most of the power comes from the triceps and some from the action of shoulder flexion and tension of the opposite pectoral muscles. At the same time, most users develop considerable sensitivity of control and can perform such delicate tasks as picking up cigar ash without breaking it. The

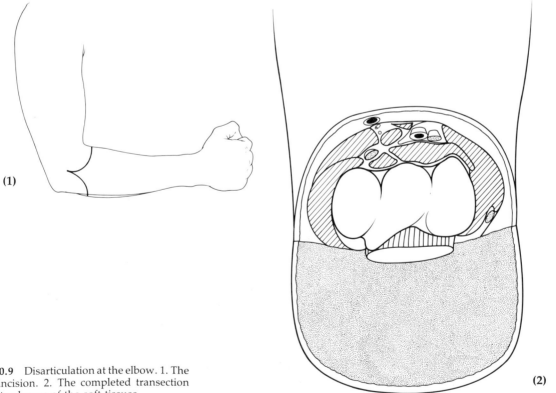

(1)

(2)

Fig. 10.9   Disarticulation at the elbow. 1. The skin incision. 2. The completed transection prior to closure of the soft tissues

forearm amputee who has sufficient motivation can perform many tasks, even those needing considerable manipulative skill.

Krukenberg's operation

A variety of operations has been devised in upper limb amputations to enlist residual function. Certain amputations of both arm and forearm are frequently unable to utilize all the muscle bellies available and since early efforts by Putti and Sauerbruch various attempts have been made to use these muscles by producing so-called kineplastic tunnels. Loops of skin are formed and muscle bellies or tendons passed through them in an attempt to produce an additional active motor, e.g. a flexor tunnel with the biceps passed through it to act as an elbow flexor in above-elbow amputations. Enthusiasm waxed and waned for such procedures in various countries but long-term problems in retaining the tunnel have resulted in almost complete abolition of these procedures, with the exception of the biceps kineplasty for operating the terminal device in forearm amputation which a few surgeons still claim has advantages.

One type of kineplastic procedure performed is the Krukenberg operation. This is rarely performed in Great Britain although it has been widely accepted in Germany. The object of the operation is to convert the radius and ulna into crocodile jaws whilst preserving a certain amount of sensation. Its real indication is for bilateral forearm amputees; some surgeons consider that it might be of value to bilateral amputees who are blind. However, all such individuals in Britain have refused the operation. It is certainly ugly and can cause psychological problems. If performed it is still possible to wear reasonably conventional prostheses as well.

Technique. The skin incision commences on the volar surface of the forearm 7 cm below the elbow joint crease to the ulnar side of the midline and is carried distally round the stump and then proximally to a point at the same level on the dorsal surface.

The incision is deepened on the volar surface, splitting the flexor digitorium sublimis into radial and ulnar portions. The flexor digitorum profundus and the flexor pollicus longus are resected entirely in order to reduce the bilk and render skin closure easier. The median and ulnar nerves are cut short but care must be taken to preserve branches to any of the remaining musculature. The interosseous membrane is divided close to the ulna for at least 12 cm. The radial portion of the flexor digitorum sublimis is sutured to the flexor carpi radialis and the ulnar portion is sutured to the flexor carpi ulnaris. The extensors of the forearm are conveniently divided into radial and ulnar groups. After fashioning the bone ends, grooves are cut in them and the radial extensors and flexors are sutured in the radial groove and the ulnar muscles in the ulnar. The ulnar portion of the incision should allow easy closure of the skin round the radius. A skin

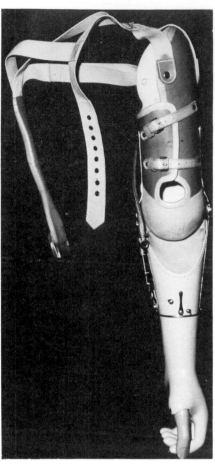

Fig. 10.10   A prosthesis for a through-elbow amputation. From W. Parry (1981), with kind permission of the author and the publishers, Butterworths

graft may have to be utilized to complete closure of the ulnar portion.

Movement should be commenced as soon as skin healing is complete. Opening of the jaws is produced mainly by the brachioradialis. Closure of the jaws is produced by the pronator teres and forearm flexors.

THE ELBOW

Occasionally the extent of the trauma or disease affecting the hand or forearm may be too great to allow a useful below-elbow stump to be fashioned. In such instances amputation above the elbow should be performed leaving adequate room for the elbow mechanism.

Disarticulation at the elbow should be avoided if at all possible. The prosthesis is bulky and cosmetically unacceptable both for men and women. The joints have to be set outside the socket resulting in excessive width at condyle level (see Fig. 10.10).

THE ARM

Amputation through the humerus

The commonest indication is severe trauma. Occasionally this amputation is necessary following sepsis or malignant tumours. As elsewhere in the upper limb the level may be determined by factors beyond the surgeon's control. The ideal is 10 cm above the elbow joint, which leaves room for the elbow mechanism in the prosthesis and provides the best length of stump for controlling an activated prosthesis. Above this level as much of the stump as possible should be retained.

Technique.
General anaesthesia and if possible a tourniquet should be used. Equal anterior and posterior skin flaps are fashioned, the skin incision commencing medially and laterally 9 cm above the medial and lateral epicondyles. The muscles are divided anteriorly and posteriorly 3 cm distal to the proposed level of bone section so that they can be sutured under normal tension to cover the bone ends. Median, ulnar and radial nerves are drawn down and sectioned so that they retract out of the wound. The vessels are ligated and the brachial artery doubly so. The humerus is divided and its cortical edges smoothed off by a file. The tourniquet is released and haemostasis is secured. The elbow flexors are sutured to the triceps expansion over the end of the humerus. The fascia and skin are sutured with interrupted sutures and the wound is drained. A wool and crêpe dressing is applied.

Amputation through the neck of the humerus

This operation does not leave the patient with any functional stump and should not be performed when it is possible to leave a humeral stump extending to three finger breadths below the anterior axillary fold. This is the critical minimal length to which an above-elbow prosthesis can be fitted. If the amputation is being performed for malignant tumour of the humerus there is no alternative but disarticulation at the shoulder joint. To leave the humeral head in situ when it is permitted on pathological grounds, however, produces a better cosmetic appearance and a more comfortable prosthesis.

Technique. No special preoperative preparation is required General anaesthesia is necessary. The patient lies on his back with a large sandbag under the dorsal spine and shoulder so that the upper trunk is rotated and tilted at about 30°.

The anterior incision extends from the tip of the coracoid

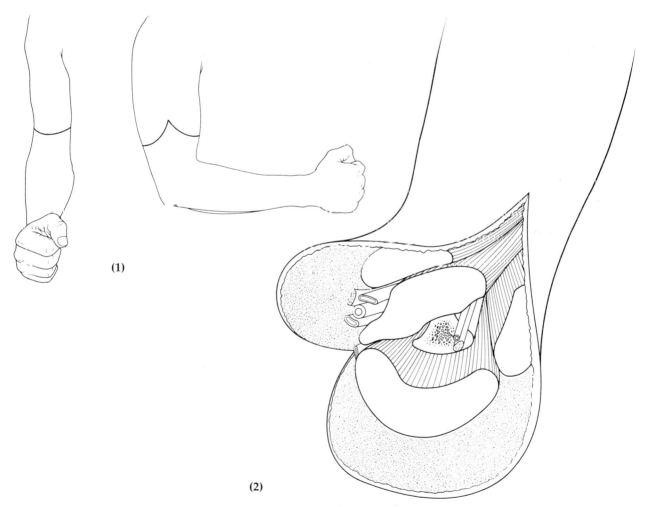

(1)

(2)

Fig. 10.11 Amputation across the lower third of the upper arm. 1. The skin incision. 2. The completed dissection prior to the closure of the soft tissues

process, downwards along the anterior border of the deltoid to its insertion and then backwards and upwards along the posterior border of the deltoid to the posterior aspect of the axilla. A vertical incision is then made joining these two points from the anterior to the posterior axillary fold across the floor of the axilla. The incision is deepened anteriorly and posteriorly. The deltoid muscle and fascia and skin are reflected upwards as a large thick flap, having dissected the deltoid free from its insertion. Anteriorly the pectoralis major muscle is divided close to its insertion and reflected medially, exposing the coracobrachialis and the pectoralis minor. The gap between these is deepened and the neurovascular bundle can be demonstrated. The coracobrachialis and the biceps are divided just below the proposed level of bone section. The axillary artery and vein are divided and doubly ligated above the level of bone section. The median, ulnar and radial nerves are drawn down into the wounds, divided cleanly and allowed to retract up into the axilla. By externally rotating the arm slightly the latissimus dorsi and teres major are easily demonstrated and divided close to their insertion into the humerus. The long head of the biceps and finally the triceps is divided about 2 cm below the base of the great tuberosity.

The humerus is sectioned at the level of its neck. The bone edges are smoothed off and haemostasis is secured. The bony stump is covered by suturing the long head of the triceps to the coracobrachialis and biceps. The pectoralis major is sutured laterally to help cover the stump and the deltoid is brought down to cover the whole of the stump. The fascia and skin are sutured in layers and a suction drain is brought out through the posterior skin flap. The wound is dressed and a crêpe bandage shoulder spica is applied.

Prostheses for humeral amputations

The highest level of amputation for the use of the range of prostheses is about 6 cm below the anterior axillary fold. Stumps shorter than this give no adequate control and a prosthesis appropriate to a disarticulation at the shoulder must be used.

The socket is made from a cast of the stump using leather or plastic. Cup-shaped inner sockets to the shape of the stump are used for short or conical stumps. The socket extends medially up to the axillary fold and laterally to the point of the shoulder. Although rotation of the humerus at the shoulder is retained it cannot be imparted to the prosthesis. In shorter stumps an extended socket is used which gives greater control of the prosthesis, although limiting abduction to some extent.

The elbow mechanism is composed of two parts. There is a simple uniaxial joint allowing flexion to 60° and extension to 180° at the elbow. Flexion is obtained passively from the other hand or actively, either by pressing downwards on the partially flexed forearm on the edge of a table or by using the flexion cord. When tensed, by rounding the shoulders or flexing the stump or both,

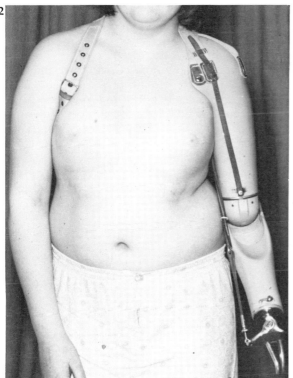

10.12

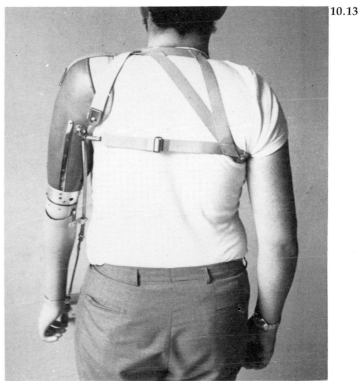

10.13

the cord will firstly flex the forearm and when locked will actuate a terminal device. In order to operate this, and to carry or push any load with the flexed forearm, the elbow must be locked. The 'automatic' elbow lock is an alternating lock operated by a lever to which is attached a strap or cord extending up to the front of the shoulder, then attached to the webbing suspension. By thrusting the shoulder forward and pulling the stump and prosthesis backwards this strap is stretched so that it pulls on the operating lever to lock and unlock the elbow joint. Alternatively, it may be used passively by the other hand.

Above the elbow joint, and its locking mechanism, is fitted a ring device to allow rotation about the long axis of the arm. The desired position may be maintained by friction or by a bolt locating into holes in the rotating ring.

Suspension of this prosthesis is by three webbing straps passing upwards from the anterior, superior, and posterior edges of the socket to meet above the shoulder. From their junction a strap passes across and below the nape of the neck to a webbing loop, which passes round the opposite axilla to provide fixation. A further strap from the same point passes across the back obliquely down to the lower part of the axillar loop. To its top is attached the strap to operate the automatic elbow lock. A further webbing strap passes horizontally from the axillar pad across the back,

Fig. 10.12 A patient wearing an immediate postoperative prosthesis after an above-elbow amputation

Fig. 10.13 Left above-elbow amputee wearing a working type prosthesis. From W. Parry (1981), with kind permission of the author and the publishers, Butterworths

where it is attached to a flexion cord. The latter passes through a pulley on the back of the socket and thence to a forward-projecting lever attached to the upper and medial part of the forearm. If actuation of split hooks, etc., is required the cord will then pass through an eye in the elbow-flexion lever to be attached to the terminal device.

The forearm of these prostheses is either made in one piece with the hand for those whose need is for a social 'sleeve filler', or a bisection and rotary is fitted either at the wrist or 5 cm (2 in) proximally.

The extent to which these prostheses are used depends upon the motivation of the patient. Bilateral above-elbow amputees have become completely independent and drive cars, play golf, etc.

THE SHOULDER

Disarticulation of the shoulder

Technique. The exposure and skin incisions are the same as for amputations through the surgical neck of the humerus. The exposed capsule of the shoulder joint is incised anteriorly and, following internal rotation of the shoulder, posteriorly. The

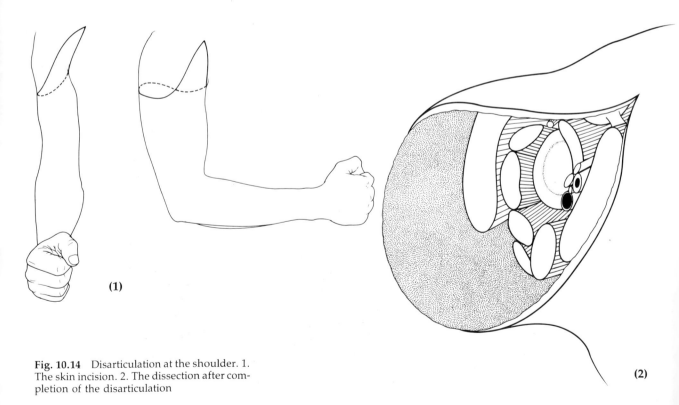

(1)

(2)

Fig. 10.14 Disarticulation at the shoulder. 1. The skin incision. 2. The dissection after completion of the disarticulation

muscles are sectioned close to their insertion and the remainder of the capsule divided to complete severance of the limb. The cut ends of the muscle are reflected into the glenoid cavity and are sutured in position. The flap containing the deltoid muscle is brought downwards and fixed below the glenoid. If the acromion is unduly prominent beneath the skin it should be partly excised to give a more smoothly rounded contour to the shoulder. The skin is trimmed and approximated by interrupted sutures. The wound should be drained.

Prostheses for shoulder disarticulation

This is one of the few levels of amputation by dislocation at a joint in which the prosthetist would not prefer a true disarticulation to a modification. A true disarticulation, which empties the glenoid fossa, leaves the acromion and clavicle projecting laterally to present a sharp angle which it is difficult to protect from trauma by a socket. An amputation through the surgical neck of the humerus maintains a rounder contour more suitable for the provision of a comfortable prosthesis and is therefore preferred.

A cast of the shoulder and upper thorax is taken and from this a shoulder cap of blocked leather is made. This extends over the chest wall anteriorly, medially and posteriorly and the upper edge is trimmed to approximately 2.5 cm medial to the acromion process. Because of the prominence of the latter, following disarticulation a large aperture is usually necessary in the top of the leather shoulder cap, which is then covered by thin Persian calf leather. This allows free movement of the acromion.

Some patients require only the shoulder cap and upper arm piece to protect the shoulder and its scar and to provide a partial sleeve filler, but the majority do require total replacement. For

Fig. 10.15 A patient after disarticulation at the shoulder. From W. Parry (1981), with kind permission of the author and the publishers. Butterworths

Fig. 10.16 The prosthesis for use after shoulder disarticulation. From W. Parry (1981), with kind permission of the author and the publishers, Butterworths

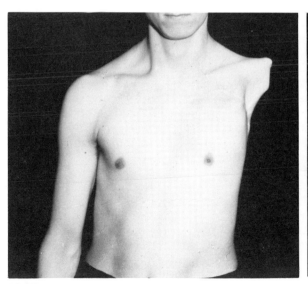

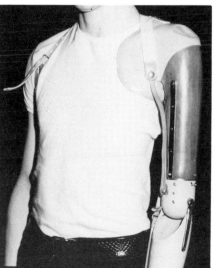

10.15

10.16

these patients the hand, forearm and elbow mechanism as supplied for a humeral shaft amputation is used, although the lock must be operated by the opposite hand as there is no shoulder control. The prostheses is held on the body by means of straps similar to those used on above-elbow prostheses.

At this level of amputation the functional activities of the artificial arm are very limited. Movement at the shoulder must largely be abandoned in favour of stability. Nevertheless, these arms are useful for steadying or holding down objects while writing, cutting, etc., and the flexed forearm can be used for carrying. There are a number of people born with complete absence of both upper limbs and experience has proved that if they have good lower limbs *no* prostheses should be fitted since the feet are capable of excellent prehension.

Forequarter amputation

This amputation is rarely performed and is indicated mainly for malignant tumours around the shoulder joint, particularly where the tumour has spread into the surrounding muscles so that the less mutilating procedures of disarticulation of the shoulder or amputation through the neck of the humerus are no longer practicable. Two standard techniques are advocated but the authors only have experience of the first of these. It may well be that the second technique, attributed to Littlewood, in which the approach is from the posterior aspects of the shoulder joint, is easier.

Technique. The incision commences at the outer border of the sternomastoid, extends laterally along the clavicle and over the acromion to the posterior aspect of the shoulder and continues along the spine of the scapula and down the vertebral border. The lower incision begins in the middle of the clavicle passing across the front of the shoulder in the groove between the deltoid and pectoral muscles and under the axilla to join the other incision at the lower angle of the scapula. The clavicular incision is deepened and the clavicle exposed by a mixture of blunt and sharp dissections. The external jugular vein may need to be divided. The clavicle is divided medially and lifted upwards and outwards towards the acromioclavicular joint. By dividing the pectoralis major muscle at its humeral insertion, and the pectoralis minor at the coracoid, the neurovascular bundle can be exposed completely. The subclavian artery and vein are dissected free and doubly ligated. The brachial plexus is divided as high up as possible and allowed to retract. Division of the latissimus dorsi and the other soft tissues anteriorly allows the arm to fall backwards freely. The arm may now be pulled forwards and downwards and the remaining muscles fixing the thorax to the scapula are divided, starting with the trapezius and extending through the posterior strap muscles at the back. The serratus anterior is finally sectioned and the forelimb can then be lifted free. The muscles remaining attached to the thorax should, if possible, be sutured together to provide some extra padding and covering over the upper and outer aspects of the thorax. The skin flaps are finally trimmed and sutured by interrupted sutures. The wound must be drained.

Alternative technique for the shoulder.
We have no personal experience of this technique which is performed basically from the posterior aspect of the shoulder and is attributed to Littlewood. Apparently the procedure can be performed rapidly and with little blood loss. Access to the vessels is considerably easier than by the anterior approach. The patient lies on the normal side of the body. The posterior incision commences at the medial end of the clavicle and extends laterally along the bone and then across the acromion process to the posterior axillary fold. It then continues downwards along the axillary border of the scapula to a point just below the scapular angle, finally turning medially to end 5 cm from the midline. The entire full-thickness flap of skin and subcutaneous tissues are dissected from the scapula and its muscles to a point just medial to the vertebral border of the scapula. The trapezius and latissimus dorsi muscles are identified and divided close to the medial border of the scapula. The levator scapulae, rhomboids, serratus anterior and omohyoid muscles are divided as the arm and scapula are gradually rotated forwards and outwards. In the upper part of the dissection the transverse cervical and transverse scapular arteries will be found and require ligation.

The clavicle is dissected free posteriorly and divided at its medial end together with division of the subclavius muscle. The upper extremity will now fall forwards, placing the subclavian

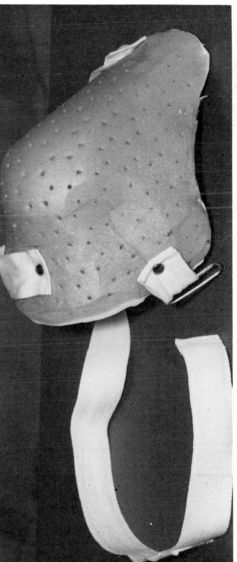

Fig. 10.17   The plastazote shoulder cap

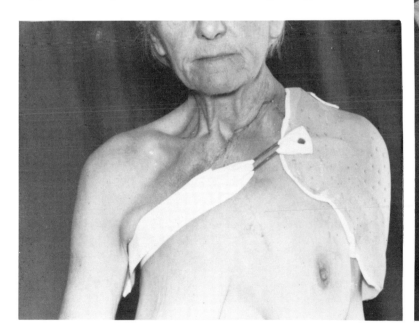

vessels and brachial plexus under some tension. The cords of the brachial plexus are divided close to their exit from the spine and the subclavian artery and vein are doubly ligated and divided. The anterior incision is now commenced at the mid-clavicular line and it curves downwards just lateral to, but parallel with, the delta pectoral groove. It crosses the anterior axillary fold and joins the posterior incision at the lower third of the axillary border of the scapula. The pectoralis major and minor muscles are divided. Haemostasis is secured and the flaps are sutured. The wound must be drained for 48 hours and a firm compression dressing is applied.

Prostheses for forequarter amputation

At this level of amputation, which is usually for malignant disease, the urgent need is for a speedy reduction in the deformity. The immediate need is for a light shoulder cap which will give the least possible pressure on the chest wall, which may be painful from its recent operation. The cap will fill up the shoulder of the clothing to give a normal outline and, particularly in women, to carry the shoulder straps of underclothing. These shoulder caps are usually made of foam plastic materials which are light and easily shaped, and supplied with a washable nylon cover.

As the patient progresses and becomes used to the weight and contact of this shoulder cap a full prosthesis cap can be manufactured. Such a limb has only a little use other than for appearance and is a dead weight to wear. Some patients, after trying it, opt to use a shoulder cap only. Whether a shoulder cap or a full prosthesis is used, it has to be held firmly to the sloping contour of the chest wall by webbing or plastic straps which encircle the chest wall. The full prostheses is otherwise similar to that supplied for a shoulder disarticulation.

11

Below-knee Amputations and Prostheses

THE FOOT

Amputation of all toes

Whilst this procedure may be necessary for extensive trauma, the usual indication is multiple toe deformities which cannot be corrected by other surgical measures. Gross hallux valgus with severe displacement of other toes and fixed flexion deformities of interphalangeal joints may be a heavy handicap, and pain, particularly from callosities under the metatarsal heads and over the interphalangeal joints, may be considerable. Often, and particularly in rheumatoid arthritis, the deformity of the toes is such that when the patient is standing none of the toes touches the ground. Comfortable footwear is almost impossible to obtain and the deformed foot and toes can only be accommodated in specially made surgical shoes with an ugly bulbous toecap.

Despite the discomfort patients are frequently reluctant to have their toes amputated and are often helped in making a decision, as with amputations at other levels, by meeting patients who have undergone this procedure

Technique. No specific preoperative measures are required apart from efforts to eliminate local infection if it exists. General anaesthesia is required and a tourniquet makes the operation simpler and quicker. The tourniquet should be pneumatic and applied above the knee. Unless applied properly, below-knee tourniquets may damage the lateral popliteal nerve as it passes round the neck of the fibula.

The raquet incisions formerly used have been superseded by equal plantar and dorsal flaps, although best use can be made of viable skin, and raquet and a symmetric flap incisions may be satisfactory. In ischaemic feet, sutures are best avoided and paper Steristrips preferred.

The metatarsal heads are always very prominent in the sole of the foot and are covered only by thickened skin and sometimes painful bursae. They should be completely excised, the bone being sectioned through the metatarsal neck just behind the head. The plantar surface in particular should be left smooth and not unduly prominent when palpated through the plantar skin. The metatarsals are cut so that they form a gently curved arc convex forwards, the second metatarsal being at the apex of the curve. If a metatarsal head remains prominent it will take an extra amount of pressure on prolonged weight-bearing and a new painful callosity will develop.

Fig. 11.1 Skin incisions for digital amputations on the foot

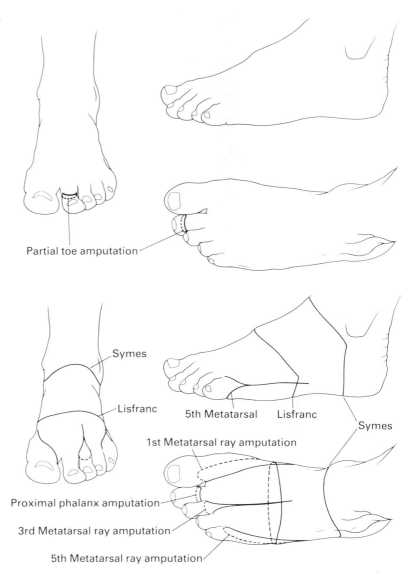

The sesamoids in the flexor tendons under the first metatarsal head should be excised. Any extruding tendons should be gently pulled down and sectioned so that they retract back from the wound. Digital nerves, not usually clearly seen because they lie between the clefts, are cut so that they too retract from the wound. Obvious vessels are ligated and haemostasis then finally secured after release of the tourniquet. Subcutaneous tissue and skin should be sutured only if Steristrips are not adequate and the scar is terminal. Drainage is not required unless there is a risk of infection.

A firm crêpe bandage is applied over a large quantity of wool

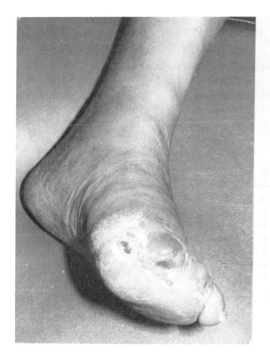
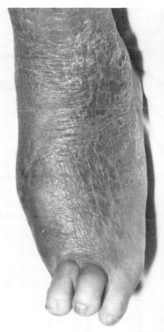
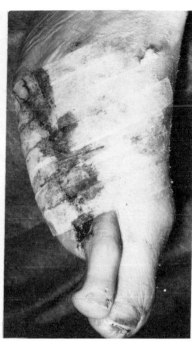

Fig. 11.2 Amputation of various toes.

and should cover the ankle as well as the foot. Unless the foot is ischaemic it must be elevated in bed for the first 48 hours after operation. Only limited dependency of the limb, and very limited weight-bearing using crutches, is allowed after this time. Sutures should be removed after 14 days but if the patient has rheumatoid arthritis and is taking steroids the sutures should be left for three weeks. After wound healing the patient can progress rapidly to full weight-bearing, wearing at first a slipper, then a shoe; no insole or foot support is usually required. Almost any type of shoe can be worn eventually. A sponge or Plastazote filler is used to occupy the space at the front of the shoe.

There is no functional loss from this operation as the toes are not amputated until they have ceased to serve any useful purpose. There is more often a functional gain, with increased ability to stand and walk in comfort.

Partial foot amputation

This operation is generally mentioned in the textbooks of surgery only because of its historical importance. The two best-known procedures are the mid-tarsal amputation of Chopart and the tarsometatarsal amputation of Lisfranc, but both have a poor reputation. The operations, as performed in the past, were almost invariably followed by severe equinus deformity due to the unbalanced activity of the calcaneus tendon. Pain from callosities and frequent ulceration over the antero-inferior aspect of the calcaneum favoured amputation at the higher level of Syme.

Fig. 11.3 Mid-foot amputations. 1. Skin incision for transmetatarsal amputation. 2. The lines of standard mid-foot amputations. 3. Structures encountered in the transmetacarpal amputation

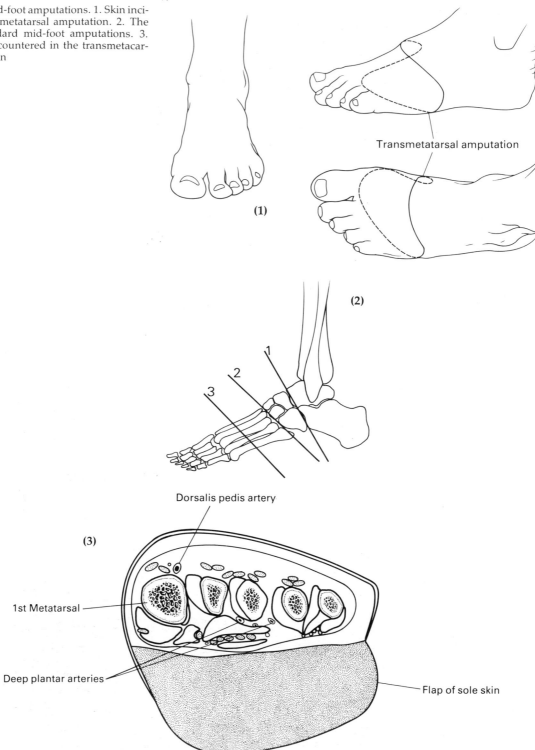

Transmetatarsal amputation

(1)

(2)

1

2

3

Dorsalis pedis artery

(3)

1st Metatarsal

Deep plantar arteries

Flap of sole skin

Whilst this is still almost universal opinion, our own experience with Chopart's amputation together with that of others, such as Bingham and Marquardt, justifies description of the procedure modified by tendon transfer to retain a balance of power in the hindfoot. The indications for the operation are rare and it is generally performed for severe injuries to the forefoot. It has no place in arteriovascular disease or cold injury.

Technique. The incision starts on the medial border of the foot, just behind the tuberosity of the navicular, and extends to the middle of the first metatarsal shaft. It runs across the sole of the foot, curving to outline a plantar flap a little longer medially than laterally. Laterally it extends to a joint just proximal to the styloid process of the fifth metatarsal. The proximal points of this incision are joined by a dorsal incision which is convex distally.

The plantar flap is dissected proximally, preserving as much as possible of the plantar fat until the talonavicular joint is exposed. Separation through the talonavicular and calcaneocuboid joint is then easily effected, manipulating the forefoot in a valgus direction and dividing all the ligaments and capsular structures. The tibialis anterior tendon should be left as long as possible and, together with the toe extensors, should be fixed firmly in a drill hole in the neck of the talus with a transfixion suture. The flexor muscles in the sole are divided and allowed to retract. The

Fig. 11.4   Through-foot amputations.

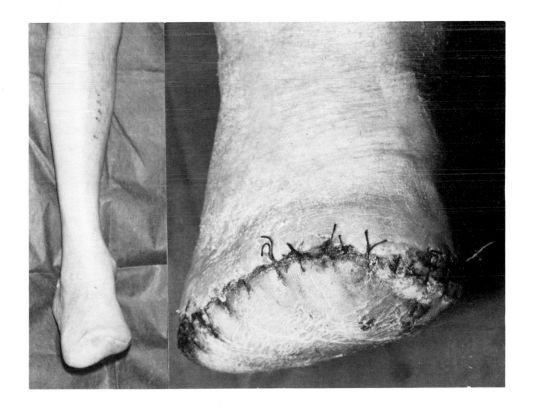

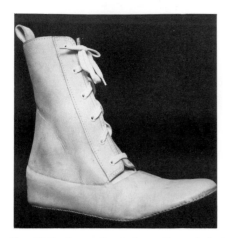

Fig. 11.5 A prosthesis for a through-foot amputation.

dorsalis pedis and plantar vessels are ligated. The flaps are finely trimmed and sutured so that the scar lies just on the dorsum of the stump. Suction drainage should be used and a padded plaster cast applied with the ankle in slight dorsiflexion. The plaster is retained for four weeks, after which weight-bearing may begin.

Syme's amputation

The technique for this operation does not differ significantly from that originally described by Syme and the numerous attempts to modify the operation have seldom succeeded in improving the end result. Opportunities to use the procedure are now relatively uncommon and as a method of choice it is often forgotten. It may, however, be the best level for amputation in chronic infections of the foot, particularly those associated with perforating ulcers and neuropathies and diabetes. Cases of leprosy, chronic foot infection, and deformities associated with myelomeningocele may be suitable provided that sensation in the postero-inferior aspect of the heel is preserved. Severe injuries to the foot, and occasionally ischaemic disease, may also be treated by Syme's amputation. It is an operation that is particularly well suited to the prosthetic management of certain severe congenital deformities of the lower limb in which the foot may be normal in appearance but useless in its function, such as is seen with a severe congenital shortening of the femur.

Provided that a good stable stump is achieved with the heel pad as the weight-bearing surface, full body-weight can be carried on the end of the stump and prosthetic requirements are therefore simplified; in countries where sophisticated prosthetic services are lacking it is ideal. The stump, provided that the skin is stable, is remarkably trouble-free and postoperative use for as long as 40 years is not uncommon. However, the conventional prosthesis is bulky, particularly over the flare of the malleoli, and it is therefore unacceptable to most women as it results in noticeable asymmetry of the ankles and calves.

Technique. No specific preoperative measures are required except eradication, if possible, of infection. An above-knee tourniquet should be used except in cases of peripheral vascular disease. General anaesthesia is used and the patient lies supine with his foot just projecting over the end of the operating table.

Two points, the first 1.75 cm below the lateral malleolus and the second 2.5 cm below the medial malleolus, are joined by a horizontal incision; a vertical incision curved slightly forwards passing across the sole of the foot at the anterior end of the heel pad is then made to join it. The vertical incision is deepened, dividing all structures in the line of the skin incision until the calcaneum is exposed on all three sides. The dorsal incision is deepened, dividing all structures at the front of the ankle joint until the ankle joint is opened to expose the neck of the talus. The foot is plantar flexed and the talus pulled firmly forwards and

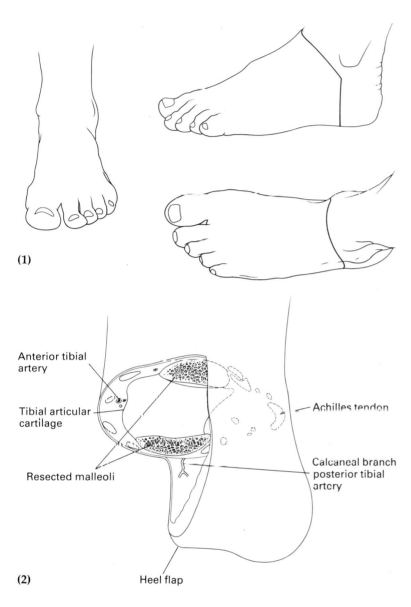

(1)

(2)

Anterior tibial
artery

Tibial articular
cartilage

Resected malleoli

Achilles tendon

Calcaneal branch
posterior tibial
artery

Heel flap

Fig. 11.6 Syme's amputation. 1. Incision lines. 2. Classical Syme's amputation after resection of the foot

downwards with a bone-hook. The capsular attachments and the medial and lateral ligaments are divided by sharp dissection and the talus gradually peeled forwards out of the ankle mortice. The superior and posterior aspects of the calcaneum gradually come into view and the Achilles tendon is divided close to the insertion into the calcaneum. Great care must be taken to keep the dissection virtually subperiosteal in order to minimize the risk of perforating the posterior heel skin, which is thin and closely adherent to the calcaneum. Pulling the foot further forwards and downwards, the dissection is continued along the inferior aspect of the calcaneum, remaining close to the bone so that virtually all of the soft tissue remains in the heel skin-flap, until the vertical incision is reached. Attention is now turned to the lower ends of the tibia and fibula and by a little dissection and retraction they can be easily exposed. After minimal periosteal stripping a transverse cut is made in the tibia and fibula with a saw 1 cm above the ankle mortice, care being taken to ensure that the cut is exactly at right angles to the plane of the leg, so that later when the patient is standing this surface will be horizontal in relation to the ground. Unless this section is horizontal, the heel pad will become unstable on standing.

The anterior and posterior tibial vessels are identified and ligated; care must be taken to preserve the calcaneal branches on which the vascularity of the heel flap depends. The anterior and posterior tibial nerves are gently pulled down, divided and allowed to retract. All the tendons are similarly pulled down and sectioned and allowed to retract away from the wound.

At this stage the tourniquet should be released and haemostasis secured. The wound is closed, using a suction drain brought out through the lateral aspect of the calf. Subcutaneous tissues are sewn together and then the skin is closed. The skin suture line always looks untidy, with large 'dog ears', as two incisions of unequal length and shape have been brought together. The temptation to trim the 'dog ears' must be resisted as essential elements of the blood supply to the heel pad are contained in them. Skin shrinkage soon occurs and they always disappear. The heel pad forms a rather bulbous mass over the lower end of the tibia. Since success in Syme's amputation depends upon this pad becoming stable and adherent to the cut surface of the tibia, it must be carefully held in position during the postoperative phase. A narrow strip of gauze dressing is applied to the suture line and the heel pad is firmly held in place by broad strips of non-stretch strapping which are applied to the upper posterior aspect of the calf and carried downwards and over the heel pad; this draws it forwards and presses it firmly against the lower surface of the tibia. The strapping is fixed to the shin. If for some reason strapping cannot be used an alternative, but less satisfactory, method is to transfix the heel flap with three Kirschner wires which must be left long and covered with corks. Orthopaedic wool and a plaster-of-Paris sheath are then applied, extending up to the tibial tubercle.

The drain is removed in 24 hours and the limb elevated for 48 hours. After this the patient may be mobilized with crutches but prolonged dependency must be avoided.

The sutures are removed on the fourteenth postoperative day. The strapping and plaster cast are reapplied and retained for a further four weeks.

The modified Syme's amputation

1   In order to improve the appearance of the Syme's stump the tibia and fibula are divided at a higher level above the flare of the

malleoli. This greatly diminishes the total load-bearing surface area and raises the pressure in Kg/cm^2 to a level greater than the stump can stand and its weight-bearing properties are therefore sacrificed.

2 Boyd amputation. After preparing a short dorsal skin flap and a long plantar flap, the talus is removed together with the rest of the foot, leaving the calcaneum still firmly attached to the heel flap. The os calcis is shortened anteriorly and then fixed into the ankle mortice and an arthrodesis is performed. This has the advantage of producing a stable load-bearing surface on which full body-weight can be carried, providing the arthrodesis is sound. The stump has the disadvantage of being very bulky and its length excludes the possibility of any form of ankle joint in the prosthesis. A protective 'elephant boot' may be worn over the stump. There may be a place for this amputation in underdeveloped communities where modern prostheses are not available. The prosthetic objections to the operation, however, are considerable.

A recent development in the use of Syme's amputation has been described, utilizing a two-stage procedure for treatment of patients with diabetic gangrene of the toes and forefoot. This procedure is exclusively for the patient with diabetic gangrene but who may also have an arterial occlusion. It is not used if the femoral pulse is absent and an absolute contraindication is involvement of the heels and skin by fissures or ulceration. The principle of the procedure is to clear the infected and diseased tissue as a first stage; a second operation six weeks later is used to form a useful amputation stump. At the first stage an incision is made anterior to the ankle joint and carried below the tips of the malleoli before encircling below the heel. Particular care has to be taken at all stages, as in other types of Syme's amputation, to preserve the calcaneal branches of the peroneal and posterior tibial nerves, and the heel skin is opposed to the anterior tibial skin by interrupted nylon sutures. The dead space that remains below the articular surfaces of the tibia and fibula is drained with a double-lumen irrigating drain and primary healing is obtained. The patient is not allowed to bear weight at this stage but mobility is fully encouraged. After a lapse of six weeks a further operation is performed in which an incision is made over each malleolus; this may be either vertical or horizontal according to the contour of the stump. Through the lateral and medial incision the malleoli are trimmed vertically to reduce the width of the stump and at the same time the protruding malleoli are removed to obtain a flat bone surface within the stump. Extensive soft tissue trimming is performed at the same time to reduce the redundant soft tissue which may otherwise become mobile on the bone end. After two weeks the stump is sound; the patient may commence weight-bearing and can be fitted with a Syme's prosthesis. This procedure is not recommended for an ischaemic foot due to atheromatous occlusion, unless a very good blood supply is available in the heel flap.

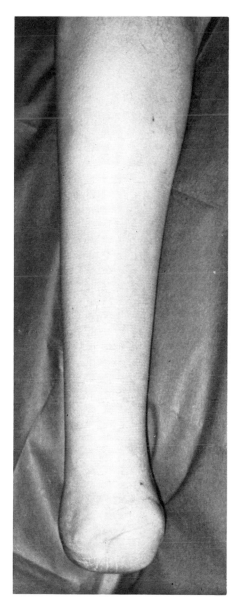

Fig. 11.7   A Syme's amputation stump.

The Syme's amputation in congenital deformities

In the modified Syme's amputation and in Syme's amputation for congenital deformities, the stump may be either end-bearing or not. When it is not end-bearing it is really a long below-knee stump, and the transmission of weight and the biomechanics are the same as in the below-knee amputation.

The modified Syme's amputation at a higher level was intended to eliminate some of the disadvantages of the Syme's amputation by making room for an ankle joint and improving the appearance by removing the malleoli. This produces problems for the limb-maker. The reduced area of the stump end increases the unit load on the end-bearing surface which is more often covered by the skin from the posterior aspect of the os calcis than the heel pad.

The majority of the modified Syme's amputations are unable to take full end-bearing and many cannot tolerate any end-bearing at all. Some of the load, sometimes all of it, must be distributed proximally, as for the below-knee amputation. The main virtues of the Syme's amputation are then lost.

The loss of the malleoli also destroys the bulbous nature of the stump. This does improve the appearance at the ankle joint but unfortunately it is then no longer a self-suspending socket and additional suspension is necessary.

When Syme's amputation is done for congenital deformities the below-knee stump is usually shorter than normal and standard prosthetic feet and ankles are supplied. The appearance of the ankle can be made cosmetically acceptable. The stump is usually not sufficiently bulbous to dispense with any additional suspension, although it may aid the suspension. In childhood these stumps may be fully end-bearing but in adult life some proximal distribution of the load, as in the below-knee prosthesis, is also usually necessary.

THE LOWER LEG

Amputation below the knee allows natural extension and flexion of the knee joint but requires a prosthetic ankle mechanism. While a long below-knee stump was advised by Silpert, and often results after emergency amputation or debridement after explosive mine injuries, this length has no advantage and patients on whom it has been performed often have a secondary amputation to provide a more conventional length so that they can be fitted with a better prosthesis.

Modern prostheses using total contact sockets with high weight loading on the tibial condyles and patellar tendon were devised in California and the patellar-tendon-bearing (PTB) prosthesis is the result; this has eliminated the need for the scar to be placed in any particular position on the stump surface. The minimum length of stump which can be fitted into a modern PTB prosthesis is 7 cm, measured down from the tibial insertion of the medial hamstring tendons. An 11 cm length of tibia is the minimum usually required. If a weight-bearing stump cannot be constructed a thigh corset and side steels must be fitted to provide weight-bearing on the ischial tuberosity. The knee joint therefore rides in a frame or socket attached to the prosthesis to provide a flexion and extension force. A spring ankle flexion mechanism is required, using a rubber cushion, a metal and rubber ball joint, or a hydraulic-controlled universal joint (Mauch joint).

The below-knee level amputation is contraindicated in any patient unable voluntarily to extend the knee joint. Uncontrolled flexion can quickly destroy the end of the stump by pressure necrosis of the tissue pressing against the bed.

A below-knee amputation transects all three muscle compartments of the lower leg. The soleal venous sinuses are transected and the calf-muscle pump mechanism is destroyed. The powerful flexor function of the gastrocnemius muscle at the knee joint is also lost.

The following major vessels must be secured: the long and short saphenous veins, the anterior tibial artery, the posterior tibial artery and the peroneal arteries together with their venae comitans. The anterior and posterior tibial nerves are also divided, together with the musculocutaneous nerve, in the peroneal compartment.

Standard technique. The classic below-knee operation is performed with the patient lying supine with the knee elevated on a large sandbag, or prone with the knee flexed. A pneumatic tourniquet is applied above the knee, unless there is ischaemic disease of the limb when a tourniquet is best avoided. The line of bone division is electively 13 cm below the knee articular surface of the tibia; 8 cm is the minimum length for a prosthesis utilizing knee flexion. Skin flaps are based on the line of bone section, the anterior being two-thirds of the limb circumference and twice the length of the posterior flap. Subcutaneous fat, fascia, and the anterior tibial periosteum are included in the flap. The saphenous veins require ligation with catgut.

The muscles, nerves, and vessels may be divided at the line of bone section, although it is an advantage if the nerves can be pulled down and then divided so that they will retract 2 to 4 cm above the line of bone section. The vessels are individually ligated with catgut, mass ligatures being avoided where possible to eliminate the remote risk of arteriovenous communication.

By upward traction with a swab between the tibia and fibula, the site of bone section is exposed and the periosteum stripped from the tibia at this site. It is easier to divide the fibula before the tibia and this should be divided 2.5 cm above the line of tibial bone section with a slight outward bevel. This is best performed with a Gigli saw or a power cantilever saw, as a bone forceps produces excessive splintering of the bone end. The anterior

Fig. 11.8 The Burgess long posterior flap below-knee amputation with gastrocnemius and soleus muscle myoplasty. 2. The structures encountered during the dissection of the long posterior flap

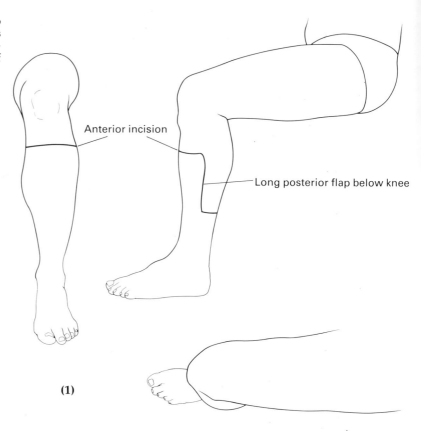

Anterior incision

Long posterior flap below knee

(1)

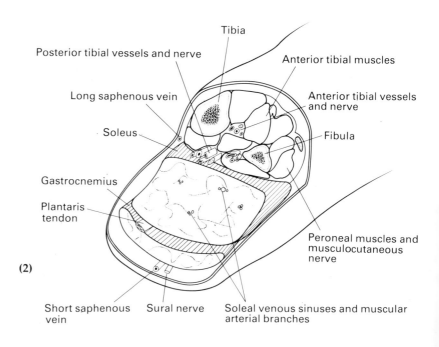

Tibia

Posterior tibial vessels and nerve

Anterior tibial muscles

Long saphenous vein

Anterior tibial vessels and nerve

Soleus

Fibula

Gastrocnemius

Plantaris tendon

Peroneal muscles and musculocutaneous nerve

(2)

Short saphenous vein

Sural nerve

Soleal venous sinuses and muscular arterial branches

bevel of the tibia is cut first by directing the saw at an angle of 45° from a point 1 cm above the line of bone section to cut through the anterior one-third of bone. The tibial section is completed by a new saw-cut from the front backwards, perpendicular to the axis of the bone at the line of bone section. The freed specimen is removed and haemostasis completed with fine catgut ligatures or diathermy coagulation. Bone wax is best avoided, and oozing from the marrow cavity soon ceases.

The skin flaps are approximated over the divided tissues by fine catgut sutures to the fascia and small nylon skin stitches or Steristrips, or by large nylon skin stitches alone. Unless there is absolute haemostasis, drainage is recommended, and suction drainage is superior to corrugated or Penrose rubber drains. A dry dressing with pressure bandage is applied unless there is a risk of sepsis. A split plaster cast adds much to the patient's comfort and aids the maturation of the stump.

Sutures are left in place for a minimum of 10 days. If nylon has been used, this time may be extended without risk of sepsis along the sutures, a useful feature in the elderly with ischaemic disease when skin healing may be very slow.

Surgical drains are removed 48 hours later or when drainage is complete.

Guillotine or circular technique. This is generally avoided as retraction of the soft tissue makes a protruding bone end and terminal scar unavoidable. It has been used in a modified form where the skin is transected well beyond the bone end, the muscles transected just distal to the bone and the bone transected at the most proximal level. This sleeve amputation allows the soft tissues to fall over the bone end, to provide skin and soft tissue cover. When this is not possible skin traction is required for two or three weeks until the soft tissues are stable on the bone end.

The sleeve amputation may have a place in the presence of severe distal sepsis but in ischaemic states the unsupported skin and subcutaneous tissue frequently become necrotic. The only recommended use for a guillotine below-knee amputation is to release a trapped victim pinned by the foot or ankle when no alternative is possible. Re-amputation is usually inevitable unless skin traction is successful in preventing retraction of the tissue.

Technique for trauma. All tissues are cleansed and full surgical debridement is performed. The bone ends are trimmed and uniform but not shaped. Skin cover is obtained using all available skin; the position of the scar and shape of the stump are of secondary importance, particularly if a total contact socket prosthesis is to be provided.

Myoplasty or myodesis is unwise at the time of injury and the aim is to obtain a healed stump, operating again later should this prove to be necessary.

Technique for ischaemia. Work with skin-dye studies has shown that the anterior skin in the region of the tibial tubercle frequently has a deficient blood supply, and necrosis of the anterior skin flap in below-knee amputations for ischaemia is frequently seen with the conventional long anterior flap. This has led to the use of equal flaps and, since the development of the total contact socket, a terminal scar is no disadvantage. The same problem has also led to the use of sleeve amputations but this does not avoid the risk of skin necrosis.

The use of a long posterior flap has been advocated and gives very good results; when combined with a limited myoplasty, this provides a stump which heals rapidly and has excellent functional results.

A transverse incision is made anteriorly 11.5 cm below the knee-joint line, extending a little over half of the circumference of the leg. The tissues are divided to the periosteum and the incision is then carried along the axis of the limb on each side for a distance of 15 cm, where a transverse incision is made around the posterior part of the circumference to form the long posterior flap. The anterior tibial muscles are divided in the line of the anterior incision and the periosteum is elevated from all surfaces of the tibia at this site. The tibia is divided with a saw 12.5 cm below the knee-joint line, the first oblique cut forming the anterior level and the second transverse cut completing the bone division. The distal fragment is steadied by a large bone-hook, inserted into the medullary cavity of the tibia while the periosteum is elevated from the fibula, which is divided with a Gigli saw, 2.5 cm proximal to the line of tibial section.

By traction on the bone-hook the posterior tibial and peroneal vessels are exposed, divided and ligated with catgut. The soleus and gastrocnemius muscles are dissected from the tibia and fibula of the specimen, which is freed by dividing these muscles at the line of the distal skin incision. The bulk of these muscles is reduced by slicing the muscle mass obliquely from the site of bone division to the end of the posterior flap. This is best performed with a Syme's amputation knife.

The cut surface of the tibia is filed smooth and all edges are rounded until the bone end is nearly hemispherical. The aponeurosis of the gastrocnemius is lifted with tissue forceps and is trimmed so that it can be sutured to the anterior tibial periosteum and the anterior tibial compartment fascia under slight tension. It is sutured with interrupted chromic catgut in this position and a suction drain or a Penrose rubber drain passed from side to side, deep to the sutured muscle. The former is brought out through the skin 8 cm above the scar.

The posterior skin flap is similarly trimmed to approximate to the anterior incision but without tension. To avoid damage to the skin, fine skin-hooks are preferred to tissue forceps. At the extremities of the flap some 'dog ear' formation cannot be avoided; care must be taken not to narrow the posterior flap in an attempt to reduce these before the skin is sutured. The sural nerve should be dissected out of the posterior flap to avoid

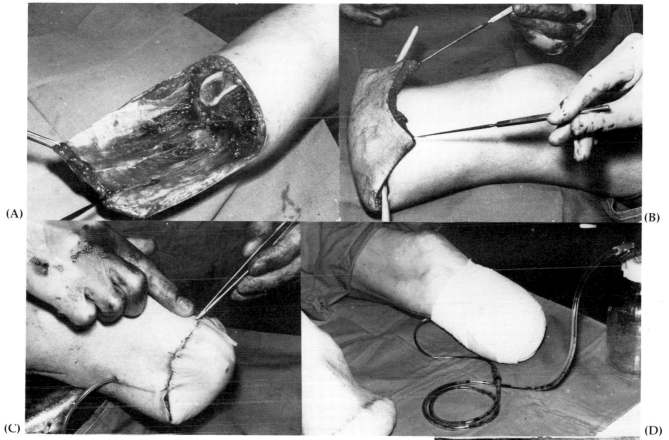

(A)

(B)

(C)

(D)

compression over the bone end.

The skin is closed with interrupted fine nylon sutures. The wound is dressed with gauze and the limb is then wrapped in a thin layer of orthopaedic cotton wool. A 10 cm wide elastic crêpe bandage is firmly applied over this, with particular care being taken to avoid a tourniquet effect proximal to the stump. The drain is removed on the third or fourth postoperative day and sutures are removed on the twenty-first day.

The long-posterior-flap procedure has the disadvantage of often resulting in a bulky stump and has to mature before it reaches an acceptable shape for socket casting. To overcome this problem the skin flaps of Tracy and Persson are combined with a myoplasty to make a skew-flap myoplastic amputation. The skin incision is made by marking the line of bone section around the leg 10–12 cm below the tibial articular surface. A point is marked 2 cm lateral to the tibial crest over the anterior compartment and a corresponding point is marked diametrically opposite on the back of the calf. A semicircle of not less than a quarter of the limb circumference in radius is described on this baseline and the line

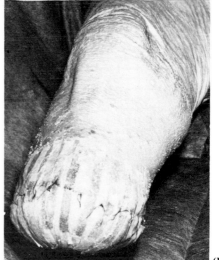

(E)

Fig. 11.9   The Burgess below-knee amputation in progress. A, Forming the long posterior flap. B, Trimming the flap. C, Wound closure with interrupted sutures and Steristrips. D, The Suction drain and bandages in situ. E, The healing stump.

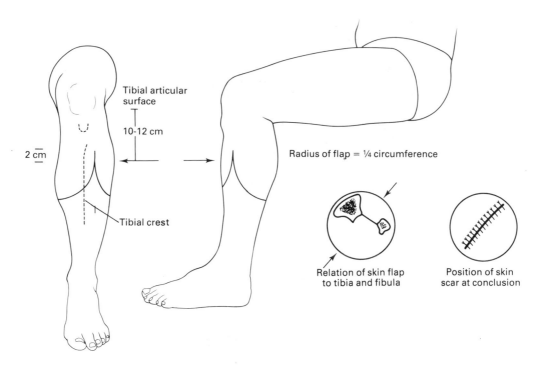

Tibial articular
surface

10-12 cm

2 cm

Tibial crest

Radius of flap = ¼ circumference

Relation of skin flap
to tibia and fibula

Position of skin
scar at conclusion

Fig. 11.10 The skew sagittal flap below-knee amputation with gastrocnemius and soleus muscle myoplasty

is extended 2 cm upward over the anterior tibial compartment. Once marked the skin flaps can be cut and thereafter the dissection proceeds as already described for the Burgess long-posterior-flap below-knee amputation. Special attention is needed to limit the width of the gastrocnemius-soleus mass so that when this is folded to form a myoplasty there will not be too much bulk in the medial and lateral aspects of the stump. The skin flaps already cut fall into place over the myoplasty and provide a parallel-sided hemispherically ended stump which will be ready for casting at an early stage.

Myodesis in below-knee amputation

When a re-amputation is necessary following trauma, or where amputation is performed as an elective procedure for an orthopaedic condition, the ability of the stump to retain full muscle function is an important consideration, and the techniques of myoplasty and myodesis have been evolved particularly in the below-knee amputation.

Below-knee amputation with a simple myoplasty for use in ischaemic disease has been described (pp 131–134). More complex soft tissue manipulations are avoided in ischaemia but can add significantly to the strength of knee flexion and venous return from the soleus muscle pump, and contractility may be preserved even in muscles which have lost their direct function.

Dederich (1963) originally sutured the anterior and posterior tibial muscles over the interosseus membrane, and the soleus–

gastrocnemius mass was sutured to the anterior tibial periosteum. A myodesis can be obtained by suturing the aponeurosis of
the Achilles tendon where it is transected to the anterior surface
of the tibia, which is drilled with three to five holes to take the
sutures. Dederich in addition now uses a bridge of periosteum
with attached bone chips between the tibia and fibula.

Part of the fibula beyond the line of the bone section may be
utilized as a transverse bone graft between the tibia and fibula.
The fibular fragment is inset into a socket cut in the tibia and this
provides a strong bridge without the introduction of foreign
materials. The square end of the stump is maintained against the
narrowing force of the socket. The free fibula segment may be
fixed between the tibia and fibula in a similar manner but a
transversely placed vitallium screw is required to secure the
bones; the screw head must be carefully countersunk and the tip
must not protrude through the tibial bone cortex. This bridge is
additionally covered by periosteum elevated from the tibia and
myoplasty of the muscle groups is performed over the bone
bridge.

Our practice is to use a bone bridge, where possible, bringing
the thinned gastrocnemius–soleus mass over the bridge to the
anterior tibial fascia and the drilled anterior surface of the tibia.
Otherwise the procedure is as that described for ischaemic disease.

PROSTHESES FOR PARTIAL FOOT AMPUTATIONS

The amputations to be considered in this section are: one or more
toes, ray amputations, transmetatarsal amputations, tarsometatarsal amputations, and midtarsal amputations.

Amputations of toes and of metatarsal rays

The loss of the great toe may interfere with the push-off at the
start of the swing phase in the more vigorous walkers, but loss of
the other digits has a minimal effect on gait. These amputations
do not require prosthetic management but the provision of a toe
filler in a normal or surgical shoe. A ray amputation can usually
be managed satisfactorily by moulding a suitable filler in either a
standard or, if necessary, a special 'surgical' shoe.

Transmetatarsal amputation

It may be possible to accommodate the remaining part of the foot
in a normal shoe with a toe filler but often a special 'surgical' shoe
is required which has a suitable 'rocker' profile and possibly a
reinforced sole.

'Tarsometatarsal (Lisfranc) and midtarsal (Chopart) amputations

Unless the surgeon has rebalanced the remaining part of the foot it will tend to go into plantar flexion and inversion, which causes many problems when attempting to fit an appliance.

If the remaining part of the foot has been rebalanced to be plantar-grade then the patient may be able to manage with an ortholene back splint incorporating a sole plate and toe filler.

If however the remaining part of the foot is plantar flexed and inverted, a 'boot-like' socket with a suitably shaped plantar pad will be required. The sole of the socket will be extended forward for the attachment of a toe filler. This type of Chopart appliance provides poor cosmesis and makes it very difficult for the patient to use normal footwear.

Fig. 11.11 A conventional blocked leather prosthesis for a Syme's amputation.

Fig. 11.12   An enclosed Syme's prosthesis.

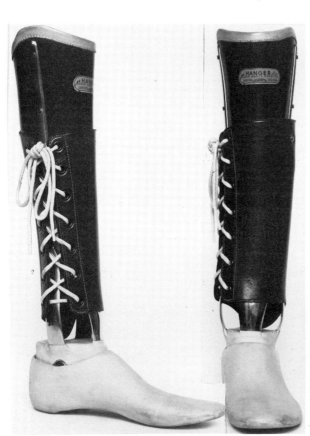

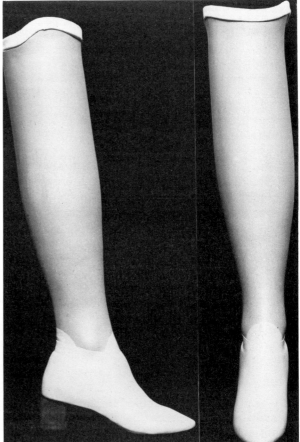

PROSTHESES FOR SYME'S AMPUTATIONS

This amputation, as described by Syme, gives a stump which is end-bearing and bulbous.

The prostheses have a resilient end-bearing pad of felt or sponge rubber on which the patient stands, taking the full body-weight during the stance phase. Because it is bulbous the artificial limb can be suspended by the stump itself. The disadvantages of the amputation for providing a good prosthesis are as follows.

1 Because the full width of the malleoli is preserved and the level of the ankle is the point of highest stress in the prosthesis, the socket and its strengthened support have to be unnaturally broad, so that the appearance is not acceptable, particularly for women.

2 Although the natural ankle-joint is destroyed by the amputation it cannot be replaced at the same level. A special ankle-joint placed below this level or a solid ankle cushion heel (SACH) foot without any ankle is used. The latter has also to be specially adapted for this level.

3 Prevention of rotation on the shaft can be difficult, particularly in children. The socket has to be moulded on either side of the anterior border of the tibia. In obese or muscular stumps, or in children who have congenital malformation, this may be ill-defined.

Temporary prostheses can be constructed of plaster of Paris, leather, or various plastics with simple peg soles often referred to as 'elephant' prostheses. More durable versions made by

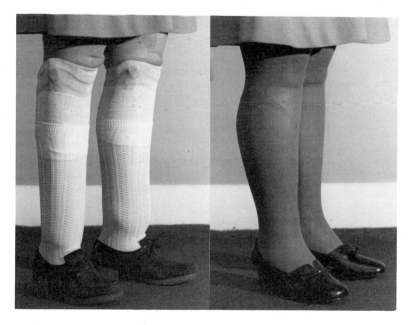

Fig. 11.13 A patient with bilateral Syme's amputations wearing conventional (left) and enclosed (right) prostheses, showing the greatly improved cosmetic result.

surgical-boot makers are very efficient 'prostheses' and are preferred by some patients. For most patients, however, they are cosmetically unacceptable and a prosthesis which is more truly an 'artificial limb' is needed.

Permanent prostheses are manufactured from leather, metal, wood or plastics according to the manufacturing techniques and skills of the country of origin.

The modern approach is to take an accurate plaster cast of the Syme's stump and on this to fashion a foam plastic liner from a material such as 'Pelite'. The re-entrant areas on the outer surface of this liner are then built up so that the liner will be able to enter a hard plastic shin which has been formed over the outside of the finished liner. The liner itself is split longitudinally over sufficient length to allow it to be drawn on over the bulbous end of the Syme's stump. When the liner with the stump in it is pushed into the hard shin of the prosthesis the split in the liner is held shut, so locking the liner and the prosthesis firmly on to the stump. It is important to re-shape the outside of the liner correctly so that the liner fits snugly into the hard shin, and yet can be withdrawn without excessive force when the patient wishes to remove the prosthesis. For a good Syme's amputation the prosthesis should be fully end-bearing with the proximal trim-line at about the upper border of the tibial tubercle. If full end-bearing cannot be tolerated the prosthesis will have to be fashioned with proximal PTB (see section on below-knee prostheses).

PROSTHESES FOR BELOW-KNEE AMPUTATION

The stump produced by below-knee amputation can be classified as long, medium or short. The length of stump can in itself be a factor in deciding upon the type of prosthesis to be used (see pages 128–129).

The prostheses are of two major types — those with artificial knee joints and side steels and those without. Prostheses without knee joints and side steels have been available for many years but were little used because neither the surgery nor the method of weight-bearing, by a plug fit, was suitable for any but a very few patients. Since 1959, when Radcliffe and Foort published the work of the University of California on the PTB below-knee prosthesis, this type of limb has become the prosthesis of choice throughout the world and is therefore described first. Prostheses with knee joints and side steels are still needed for a minority. They have many variations and only the principal varieties are described.

Patellar-tendon-bearing below-knee prosthesis

Commonly referred to as the PTB limb, this prosthesis depends upon an accurately fitting socket and even more on a correct alignment. The vertical load of weight-bearing is taken:

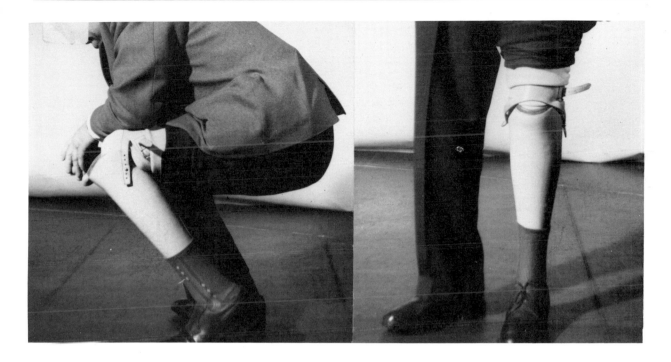

1 on the skin covering the patellar tendon. This area is covered by integuments designed for kneeling and is the natural place for applying force as in breaking sticks or bending bars. This is the major weight-bearing area

2 over a wider area under the medial tibial condylar flare

3 on a partial end-bearing

Mediolateral stability is provided by pressure on the lateral aspect of the stump and under the medial tibial condyle. Antero-posterior stability is provided by support on either side of a V-shaped groove (which protects the crest of the tibia) together with a broad area of support just distal to the popliteal crease.

The below-knee amputation stump has subcutaneous bone which will inevitably give rise to intolerably high pressures if allowances are not made by (a) giving room for these bony prominences and (b) compressing the soft tissues to some extent. A socket made to a simple cast of the stump is therefore not suitable. The case of the stump is taken in about 10–12° of flexion. During the taking of the cast some modification is made by the hands of the prosthetist to outline the patellar tendon and to provide a counter pressure posteriorly. The positive male cast has marked on it, by direct transfer of copying pencil, the areas of bony prominence. These areas are built up to a predetermined depth. The area over the patellar tendon is cut away to about 1.75 cm in depth and 4.25 cm in width. Also modified by reduction are areas under the medial tibial plateau, on either side of the anterior edge of the tibia, and over the fibula between its head and cut end. Care must be taken when smoothing out the finger marks

Fig. 11.14 A patient wearing a patellar tendon bearing prosthesis after below-knee operation.

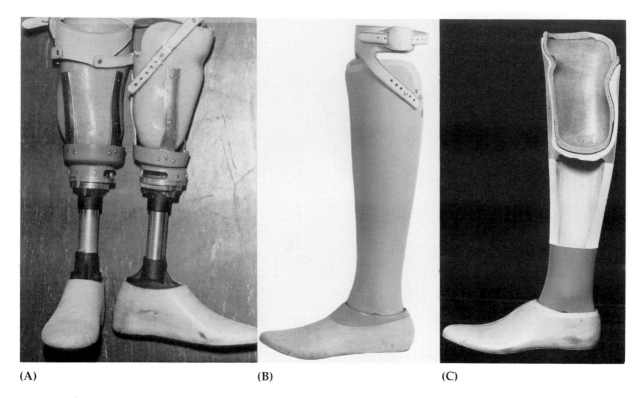

(A)   **(B)**   **(C)**

Fig. 11.15 Patellar tendon bearing prostheses for below-knee amputations. A, Modular system with alignment devices. B, C, Conventional prosthesis, exterior view and vertical section.

over the posterior area of the cast not to remove the prominences made by the hamstrings. Indeed, a slight build-up on the cast for the hamstring is sometimes made. The socket is fabricated on the modified cast using a foam plastic inner liner and a rigid plastic external socket.

The socket is then attached to an alignment device on the prosthetic foot and ankle. Correct alignment is most important with this prosthesis and an understanding of the forces acting on the stump, and how alignment can modify these forces, is necessary.

1 The socket is set in 5–7° flexion. This is the normal flexion in a knee joint in the mid-stance phase when walking and also allows the patellar-tendon bar to engage the patellar tendon with less shear.

2 The socket is positioned relative to the foot and ankle. If it is too far over the toe-break it makes the limb unstable; if it is too far over the back the knee tends to hyperextend in the stance phase, causing excessive pressure by leverage on the patellar tendon. The original description of this limb specified the incorporation of a SACH foot.

The socket is placed in this alignment so that the vertical load line when standing still falls between the anterior two-thirds and the posterior one-third of the foot. If a uniaxial foot and ankle with heel and instep rubbers is used, the socket, still with its 5–7° flexion, should be a little further back or it will unduly compress the instep rubber. The final adjustment of the socket is made using an alignment device after observing the patient walking. There are a number of such devices in use. All have to be capable of adjustment to the tilt of the socket in any direction relative to the vertical and of changing the relative position of the socket to the foot without altering the angle.

When the alignment of the prosthesis is satisfactory, the device is fixed. In many systems of modular central strut construction the device may be left in situ, but in those using stressed skin construction it is necessary to put the limb into a jig. This maintains the relative position of socket and foot, and allows the alignment mechanism to be removed and replaced by a shin (shank).

In walking with this prosthesis there is a changing pattern of pressures on the stump. In the swing phase, initially, after toe-off, the stump extends to swing the prosthesis forward. The inertia of the prosthesis tends to make it lever off the posterior rim of the socket and develop high pressure anteriorly on the distal end of the stump. At the end of swing phase the prosthesis is decelerated, largely by the hip extension, causing pressure on the patellar tendon and on the posterior aspect of the stump distally.

For the first 5° of the stance phase the pattern of distal and proximal pressure continues but after heel-strike the rotation of the foot and shin (shank) tends to produce knee flexion and the weight is transferred to the posterior proximal socket and the tibial tip anteriorly. At the same time there is vertical loading on the patellar ligament and other load-bearing areas, directed slightly backwards because of the forward motion of the body.

At toe-off one might expect this pattern to reverse but in the correctly aligned limb it does not, because knee flexion should have been motivated by the hip flexors. It is a sign of excessive instep resistance if at toe-off the patient gets excessive pressure on the patellar ligament.

The mediolateral position of the foot in relation to the socket is also important in the stance phase. The body-weight is medial to the socket. There is some inertia of the body as it sways towards the amputated side but stability has to be given to the stump in the socket by medioproximal and laterodistal pressure.

If the prosthetic foot is placed too far laterally the body weight will tend to collapse medially, resulting in gaping on the inner side of the socket and pressure on the fibular head. If placed too near the midline the pressure over the cut end of fibula and the medial tibial condyle becomes excessive and there is gaping laterally on the proximal rim of the socket.

Discomfort may arise from the use of an artificial limb when sitting. With the PTB limb there are no mechanical knee joints so there are no problems arising from the discrepancy between the human and artificial joints.

In standing it is desirable to keep the posterior wall of the socket high so as to provide a counterpressure to hold the stump onto the patellar bar. The insertion of the hamstrings is very variable but is always below the level of the tibial plateau. A common fault in making the sockets is to have a horizontal trim line to the posterior wall. This may give rise to pressure in the hamstrings when flexing the knee in walking and will certainly give rise to excessive pressure in sitting, causing the stump to come partially out of the socket.

There are also many uses of the foot in the sitting position, of which driving a car is probably the commonest. In lifting the prosthesis with the partially extended knee, gravity causes it to try to rotate round the posterior rim, a rotation which is prevented by anterior distal pressure.

Such, therefore, is the standard PTB socket and the forces which its use causes on the amputation stump. The understanding of these forces explains why the tibia should be rounded and the fibula shortened, why myoplasty is preferred by the prosthetist, and why good skin with non-adherent scars is necessary in critical areas. Apart from these areas the skin can be of quite poor quality. Indeed, even many First World War casualties who had stumps with very badly scarred adherent skin were greatly improved by conversion to PTB limbs. However, not all stumps are entirely satisfactory on PTB limbs. This is usually due to faulty manufacture of the socket and faulty alignment but is sometimes due to inherent difficulties. There are at the present time a number of modifications to the socket. Some of these are essentially in connection with suspension of the limb, yet to be discussed, but others are intended to overcome these difficulties.

The first problem is that in this, as in all prostheses, a rigid or nearly rigid socket is being fitted over bone with soft tissue interposing. Inevitably there is some piston action of the skeleton within the soft tissues as weight is put on to the amputation stump. If this pistoning is minimal and there is enough soft tissue cover, all will be well; but if the pistoning is excessive or there is little soft tissue cover, the pressure may be excessive on the end of the stump or traction on adherent scars may be intolerable.

In the original socket it was intended that there should be partial end-bearing. The periosteo-osteomyoplastic amputation with its long posterior flap provides enough soft tissue within the stump itself to give tolerance between the bone and the socket; but the standard amputation, particularly in the thin bony patient, leaves the cut end of the tibia subcutaneous, however well rounded it may be, and this cannot tolerate any end-bearing on the stump. In practice, therefore, few of these sockets are in terminal contact with the stump. This can be seen by inspecting evidence of wear on the walls of the socket; the bottom will be unmarked except for a dusting of wool powder from the stump socks.

There are inevitably circumferential pressures arising over the whole of the stump from the use of this socket. When these are intermittent, as in walking, little harm occurs, but in those who stand for long periods they progressively impede the venous and lymphatic return and over the years give rise to terminal peau d'orange, eczema, etc. Some terminal pressure is therefore desirable to assist the venous and lymphatic return. In practice in the standard PTB socket, even when it is not in contact with the end of the stump, there is a small element of pneumatic pressure that occurs during walking before air can escape past the stump. That this is effective was shown when valves were incorporated in some sockets made in the United Kingdom, to help ventilate the socket. A number of patients who had previously been trouble-free then developed terminal congestion.

However, terminal congestion will ultimately occur in a few patients. It is therefore desirable to produce a socket which has a soft end-pad that remains in contact with the stump when it is not load-bearing and which is compliant to the pistoning of the bone within the stump.

An alternative type of socket is also used in suitable cases in some centres. It is suggested that soft liners such as rubber or foam plastic distort and spoil the fit and that if a socket fits perfectly and the distribution of the load is correct, the socket can be hard with no liner. This type of fitting demands impeccable forming and a stump which has no fluctuation in size in order to avoid excessively high pressures on bony points.

Suspension of the prosthesis. The suspension of an artificial limb presents problems of comfort and interference with the rest of the body. Ideally suspension should be by the stump itself. The PTB limb is not suitable for a bulbous stump and cannot use such a stump for suspension. Attempts are being made in a number of centres to produce 'suction' socket limbs, but without any great success.

The original method of suspension described by Radcliffe and Foort was by a cuff around the thigh just above the patella, from which lateral and medial straps run obliquely backwards to studs on the socket. The purpose of the straps is two-fold: firstly to suspend the prosthesis from the patellar and femoral condyles in the swing phase and secondly to check hyperextension of the knee when standing. The positioning of the lateral and medial straps and their studs is critical if either of these functions is to be satisfactory. The cuff itself need not be tight, its purpose largely being to prevent it slipping off the patellar and femoral condyles. However, in patients with well-developed quadriceps this may be impossible and a supplementary suspension of a webbing waist-belt and an elastic pick-up to the cuff suspension is used.

An alternative suspension for women is a specially woven strong elastic stocking which is pulled over the whole prosthesis and up to the patient's own suspenders. It gives good appearance and excellent suspension for all but the most vigorous users. Its only disadvantage for most women has been the abandonment of suspenders since the introduction of tights.

But the ideal of suspension by the socket itself is still being attempted. Two methods are in use. The first, introduced by Fajal in France, is to extend the socket upwards to include the patellar

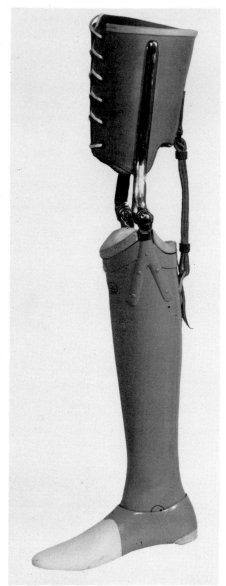

Fig. 11.16 A conventional below-knee prosthesis with corset and side steels

and the femoral condyles laterally. This extension is indented over the top of the patella and thus suspends it. As in the standard socket the cast is taken with 30° flexion. In standing, therefore, with the knee in extension, the socket can give excessive pressure above the patella. In sitting with a knee flexed to 90° there is a tendency for this socket to stand out from the normal contours. These effects are variable in different patients and this method of suspension has proved satisfactory for many.

The other method of using the socket for suspension is the 'supracondylar-wedge-type socket'. In this the lateral medial walls of the socket are extended upwards above the femoral condyle. The lateral wall curves in above the lateral femoral condyle. The cast is adjusted so that the medial wall will allow the introduction of the stump and femoral condyles into the socket. A wedge is then inserted into the medial side of the socket to lock it above the medial femoral condyle. Success is reported with this suspension but the manufacture and location of the wedge is critical if the prosthesis is to stay on in normal usage or if excessive pressure on the condyle is to be avoided. A variation on the supracondylar wedge is to make the socket wings flexible enough to spring over the femoral condyles and hold the prosthesis on the stump.

Below-knee prostheses with knee joints

The PTB limb and its variants without side steels and artificial knee joints is the prosthesis of choice for the majority of patients with below-knee amputations, but side steels, knee joints, and a high corset may be used for a number of reasons which may be justified or not. They are not added to PTB prostheses in the United Kingdom but may be elsewhere.

The reasons for adding side steels with knee joints and corsets are:
1   *Surgical.* A wrong choice of level of amputation in which the stump, while surviving, is a prosthetic embarrassment and the load-bearing and control has to be at a higher level.
2   *Prosthetic.*
  (a) To correct or attempt to correct an ill-aligned PTB limb.
  (b) To suspend a PTB limb when a correctly adjusted cuff suspension would suffice.
  (c) Because 'I always fit side steels and corset to bilateral amputees'.

Other reasons for using side steels, whether on PTB limbs or other types, are:
1   To suspend a PTB or other limb in certain occupations. Even a properly adjusted cuff suspension will not hold the limb on if the worker is walking in clay.
2   To provide stability in an unstable knee joint, whether the instability is ligamentous or muscular. The side steels and the

corset can then be used on an amputated limb as a knee cage or calliper would be used on the non-amputated limb. A ring catch or other locking device can be added to the knee joint in flaccid or spastic paralysis.

3   To redistribute and reduce the pressures developed by the moments created in maintaining stability in the stance phase of walking.

4   To provide partial or total weight-bearing at a higher level while retaining the knee joint and its musculature as a knee control mechanism. Painful arthritis and partial anaesthesia are examples in which this occurs. It may also be necessary in conditions where the patellar tendon is inadequate for weight-bearing. This is not infrequent in congenital deformities when the patella may be small and its tendon lax. It also occurs in amputations when there is a long-standing paresis with a high-riding patella and, of course, in the rarity of a below-knee amputation in a patient who has suffered patellectomy.

When artificial knee joints are introduced into the prosthetic system where the natural knee joint is also present, discrepancies between the movements of the two must be kept to the minimum by positioning the artificial joints accurately. Even then there will be relative movement between the artificial and the real limb segments. This can be reduced to some extent by using polycentric joints, but unfortunately these, while clinically an improvement on simple uniaxial joints, are mechanically less robust and tend to become loose and noisy despite remaining safe. Even so, the relative movement has to be taken up by either a loose fitting socket or a loose-fitting corset, or both. The positioning of the uniaxial joint for the PTB limb is posteriorly and above the average anatomical centre (Radcliffe and Foort, 1961). When joints are added to a PTB limb the fit of the socket is so intimate that it would be difficult to sit without some yield in the thigh corset to accommodate the relative movement. In the United Kingdom when thigh corsets and side steels are needed, the older type of limb with either a wooden socket or a block leather slip socket is used, as is common practice in North America, continental Europe, and elsewhere.

These sockets are proximal-bearing or non-weight-bearing and are usually open-ended. The wooden sockets are an integral part of the wooden shin (shank) and are carved out of it by the craftsmen. They are made to fit around the upper half of the stump from approximately 3 cm below the lower pole of the patella. The accuracy of fit depends upon the skill of the craftsman. When well made, particularly with a fleshy stump and in children, they can give trouble-free service without a blemish on the stump. In the majority of patients with this type of socket, their protestations of comfort are belied by the evidence of past and present excoriation and hyperkeratization on the stump.

The slip socket is made by blocking leather on to a cast of the stump which has been lengthened by the addition of plaster. This leather socket is then placed into the shin (shank) of the prosthesis which may be made of wood, metal, fibreglass, or other suitable material. The upper half of the socket made to the cast of the stump will also mould itself accurately to the contours of the stump in use. When the patient sits, the stump is withdrawn and displaced posteriorly so that it is lying obliquely to the shin (shank). The slip socket should move partly or wholly with the stump so that it tilts in its container, thus protecting the stump from some of the trauma of the less precise fit. Elastic straps are sometimes added from the thigh corset to the slip socket so that it will remain firmly in contact with the stump in walking and sitting.

Prosthetic corsets

The material, length, and fit of the thigh corset should depend upon the function required of it. Leather is the usual material, although various flexible plastics have also been tried. When the corset is being used only to maintain side steels in place, for stability, or to suspend the limb as used with the PTB device, it should be soft and compliant. It need then extend only about three-quarters of the way up the thigh.

The sockets of artificial limbs for below-knee amputations which are not PTB limbs are rarely used to support the total body-weight and in many patients take little or no weight. The weight is then taken partly or wholly on the high and/or ischial tuberosity and buttock. If the patient takes weight on the thigh using a soft corset, it is used with progressive tightening which leads to excessive atrophy of the musculature, a roll of flesh over the top of the corset, and possibly the formation of epidermoid cysts. If, therefore, an element of weight-bearing on the thigh is required, a stiff corset of blocked leather or similar material should be used extending up to the groin.

When the patient cannot use the stump for weight-bearing, from excessive pathology in either the stump or the knee joint, it is necessary to take the full weight proximally on the ischial tuberosity and buttock as well as the thigh. Even the long blocked leather corset then needs to be excessively tight to carry along the body weight on the thigh. The top of the corset has to be shaped to resemble the socket rim of the prosthesis for the mid-thigh amputee to ensure ischial weight-bearing. This is usually fabricated out of the same material as the corset and is suitably reinforced. It is then called a blocked leather tuber bearing corset. This, like all the other corsets described hitherto, opens down the front and is closed by lacing straps, etc. Even then the patient may be tempted not to adjust the corset correctly and the metal or plastic closed rim resembling the above-knee socket may be used. This is not in common use but is needed sometimes in senile patients, for the very obese, and on those occasions when the choice of amputation level has not been judicious.

Suspension

These corseted limbs are usually suspended by a single brace going over the opposite shoulder. This is attached to an elastic, placed posterolaterally to the top of the corset, and to an elastic crotch strap (kick strap) fixed to the top of the shin (shank). Used over a long period of time this single brace tends to produce a scoliosis. It also impedes the use of the arm in many manual occupations.

A waist-belt suspension which also has the back lift and crotch strap (kick strap) is better, but the abdominal obesity of many middle-aged and elderly amputees as well as concurrent intra-abdominal conditions often makes this unsuitable and shoulder suspension is necessary. Many then use a semi-double brace running over both shoulders and connected at a higher level with a light webbing belt. This suspends the limb and distributes its weight over both shoulders.

There are also a number of wearers, usually those who have had amputations earlier in life, who are able to suspend the limb by the corset alone. This is easier to achieve if the anterior distal border of the corset is trimmed to fit closely to the upper pole of the patella. Sometimes this may be achieved by using an excessively tight corset but many can remove the artificial limb and replace it without undoing the lacing. Of all patients these show the least wasting of the thigh.

Sitting
Sitting, even with accurately placed uniaxial joints, gives rise to undesirable pressures on the stump. The artificial joints should be placed approximately at the junction of the posterior third with the anterior two-thirds, somewhat above the level of the mean knee-joint axis. Even so, there is a tendency for the stump to be withdrawn by the thigh corset upwards and backwards relative to te socket.

Influence of stump length on choice of prosthesis

Stumps longer than 15 cm in length, unless they are done by one of the myoplastic techniques, are terminally thin with little soft tissue cover between the skin and bone. The longer stumps also are covered by skin which has a poor vascular supply. Unless a myoplastic technique has been used, few of these stumps can tolerate even the softest of end-bearing materials. In PTB limbs these stumps are subjected to circumferential pressures over almost the whole length. Without end support, terminal congestion with its consequences is therefore common and one element of weight-bearing is eliminated to the detriment of the amputation.

These long stumps, therefore, may need to be given side steels and thigh corsets so that partial or even total weight-bearing is taken above the knee joint, relieving the stump from weight-bearing in the socket and lessening the circumferential pressures. The artificial knee joint then produces its own problems, for the long lever of the stump exaggerates the difference between the real and artificial joints. It becomes increasingly difficult to protect the cut end of the tibia from excessive pressure, both in the swing phase and sitting.

The long stump will also often make it difficult for the limb-maker to give a good appearance. In men this is not usually of any great significance, but it may be a considerable cause of dissatis-faction in women. At the knee level there is the normal transverse diameter of the bone and soft tissues. This is increased in the artificial limb by the addition of the socket and its supporting material, whether this is a PTB limb or the older conventional limb. When the stump is not overlong it is easy to shape the artificial limb to match the natural limb, but when the stump is long this may not be possible.

With the exception, therefore, of the longer periosteo-osteomyoplastic operations, many prosthetists prefer that the below-knee stump should not be longer than 14 cm from the medial tibial plateau. Bone section at a higher level than this will still give excellent stumps providing there is a long enough lever to control the prosthesis. This lever depends not so much on the length of the tibial remnant as on the length below the insertion of the hamstrings and the bulk of the stump. This insertion is variable. Three fingerbreadths below the insertion of the medial hamstring are needed, although two fingerbreadths are occa-sionally sufficient. When the below-knee stump is shorter than this, the stump cannot be used effectively in any prostheses and a kneeling prosthesis must be used. This was, of course, the classic method of using the peg-leg of antiquity. The prosthesis then resembles the limbs used for disarticulation at the knee and its mechanics are similar. The short below-knee stump, fitted in this way, has some disadvantages for the prosthetist compared with the good disarticulation at the knee. In the latter, the patella lies anteriorly to the femoral condyles through which most of the weight is transmitted, the lower pole of the patella and its ligament contributing to the load-bearing surface. In the kneeling below-knee stump, the patella is pulled into an antero-inferior position and the weight is not transmitted directly to the femoral condyles. There is a much greater load on the patella itself and on its ligament, the rest of the load falling upon the tibia. A bursitis is much more likely to arise, for in use there is reflex movement in the knee joint which the prosthetist cannot eliminate. This move-ment can also cause friction on the socket at the end of the stump.

The socket, structure, and suspension of this limb are the same as that for disarticulation at the knee (see pages 157–159).

12

Through-knee Amputations and Prostheses

Through-knee amputation is not widely practised, and in many centres would be considered at least controversial, but it deserves a better reputation. It used to be practised widely but because of its ugliness and the difficulty in fitting a prosthesis it became unpopular. The fact that it is a quick and silent amputation makes it especially suitable for the sick elderly patient having the operation under spinal or epidural techniques of anaesthetic. Blood loss is minimal and it is the least traumatic of any major lower-limb amputation. More recently its special merits have encouraged its wider use; these include its strength and end-bearing properties, the retention of proprioception, its durability and shape which favour retention of a prosthesis, together with the possibility of early fitting associated with advances in prosthetic design. It is in every sense preferable to an above-knee amputation and in the elderly, in whom amputations for ischaemic disease are common and often eventually bilateral, the chances of achieving satisfactory ambulation after bilateral through-knee amputation is much greater than with above-knee amputation. Patients can, moreover, be independent over limited distances without prostheses and can walk adequately on short pylons even if they fail to cope with formal length prostheses. The main contraindication to through-knee amputation is a severe flexion deformity at the hip joint.

The standard operation in the past was performed with a long anterior flap, the blood supply of which in arteriovascular disease was often tenuous, resulting in a significant but generally acceptable rate of failure. Recently the operation has been modified by the utilization of flaps based medially and laterally and the results have been significantly better. Our experience with this method, however, is not yet sufficient to justify abolition of the standard technique. It should also be noted that increasing success with the Burgess type of below-knee amputation with the long posterior flap may, by making it possible to preserve the knee joint, greatly diminish the number of candidates for through-knee amputation in the future; if ischaemia is more extensive, then above-knee amputation will have to be accepted as the alternative.

Standard technique

The operation is best performed with the patient lying prone (this approach gives better access to the structures in the popliteal fossa). The leg should lie on a 15 cm block, placed under the

Fig. 12.1 Through-knee amputation using the conventional long anterior flap. 1. The incision line. 2. Posterior dissection completed with transection of the vessels and hamstring tendons

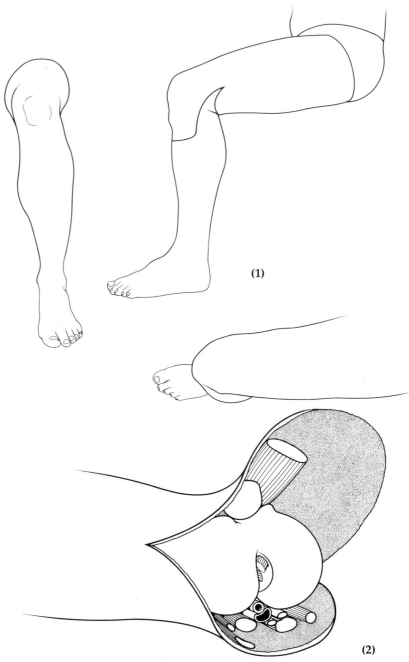

(1)

(2)

mid-thigh. A tourniquet is used only in cases with normal vascularity.

The shape of the anterior flap is vitally important. It must be as broadly based as possible, as success or failure in this operation usually depends solely on the blood supply to this flap. If it is cut too much on the curve then necrosis will occur at the tip of the flap. The flap extends for 7.5 cm below the knee joint and parallel to it, extending just over half the circumference of the leg. Each end of the incision is taken back to the knee joint. The posterior incision is 2.5 cm below the posterior knee-joint line. Both flaps are elevated with the deep fascia to expose the joint line. With the knee fully flexed the ligamentum patellae is detached from its insertion into the tibial tubercle and dissected back to the knee-joint line. The anterior capsule and synovial membrane are cut transversely and as far laterally as possible. The cruciate ligaments are severed from their tibial insertion, leaving them as long as possible. The knee is now extended. The gastrocnemius muscle bellies are divided near their origin from the lower end of the femur and the hamstrings are divided just below the knee-joint line. The vessels can now be dissected free, doubly ligated and divided, and the medial and lateral popliteal nerves gently pulled down and divided. The posterior capsule and remaining tibial attachments of the capsule are divided and the amputation is complete. If a tourniquet has been used it should be released at this stage. In cases where the viability of the anterior flap is in doubt it must be carefully inspected at this stage to see whether it is bleeding from the cut edge; if not, the amputation will have to be converted into an above-knee amputation. The patellar tendon is sutured to the cruciate ligaments, which stabilizes the patella. The hamstrings also are sutured to the cruciate ligaments, thus helping hip extension and avoiding a flexion deformity at the hip joint. The synovial membrane should be left undisturbed and no attempt should be made to remove it. The wound is closed in layers, synovial membrane and capsule together, then the deep fascia and finally the skin. The suture line should lie transversely on the posterior aspect of the knee joint just above the weight-bearing area. Suction drainage is utilized for 24 hours and a bulky loose dressing is applied. Wound healing can be expected in 14 days. An effusion may appear in the knee joint and occasionally needs repeated aspiration. Should skin necrosis occur in the adult, shaving of the condyles to effect secondary skin closure is unlikely to be successful and an above-knee amputation usually has to be performed. Weight-bearing in a pylon can start as soon as wound healing is complete. Early fitting of the definitive prosthesis is usual because there is very little stump shrinkage.

The procedure using lateral flaps is considered by many to be preferable, especially for the ischaemic patient who can only lie supine under regional anaesthetic. The skin flaps must be generous and not tight over the condyles. The lateral flaps extend for 7 cm below the medial and lateral joint lines starting anteriorly at the tibial tubercle and extending posteriorly to 1 cm below the posterior joint line. The deep fascia is dissected up with the skin to expose the knee joint and the rest of the procedure is as for the standard operation. The suture line eventually lies in the intercondylar region of the femur and usually gradually draws up posteriorly, well away from the weight-bearing area.

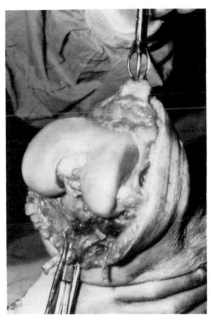

Fig. 12.2 A through-knee amputation in progress. The lateral flaps have been drawn back, and the patellar and hamstring tendons are held prior to their attachment to the cut cruciate ligaments

Fig. 12.3 Saggital flaps for through-knee amputation. 2. Exposure of the cruciate and lateral ligaments of the knee joint prior to division

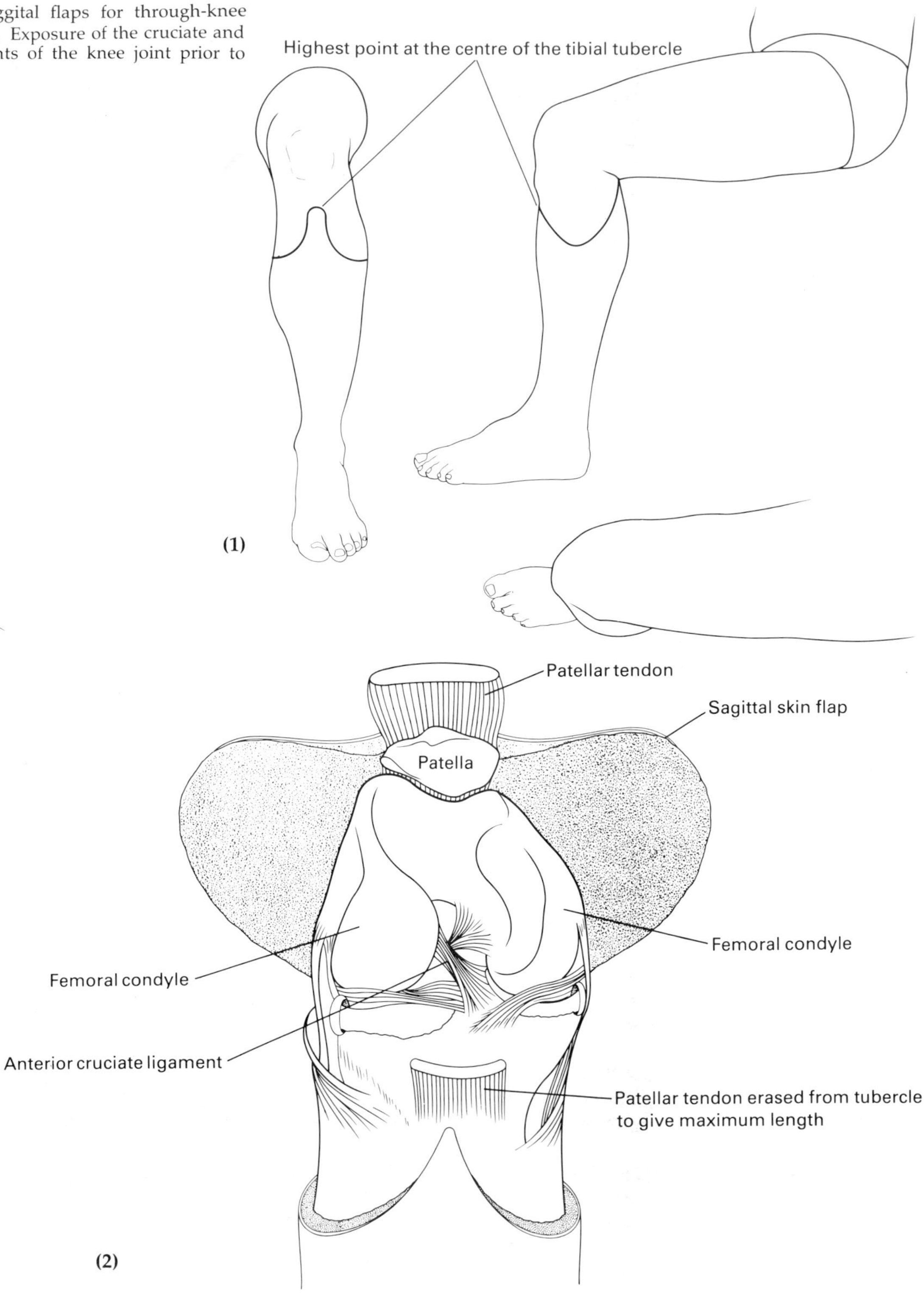

Highest point at the centre of the tibial tubercle

(1)

Patellar tendon

Sagittal skin flap

Patella

Femoral condyle

Femoral condyle

Anterior cruciate ligament

Patellar tendon erased from tubercle to give maximum length

(2)

Amputations through the distal femur

In ischaemic disease, the level of amputation is decided by consideration of the ready healing obtained at the above-knee level balanced by the realization that amputation at that level carries a higher mortality and a diminished chance of rehabilitation. Faced with this dilemma it is not surprising that intermediate levels of amputation have been used to obtain the advantages of both.

Through-knee amputation has been considered but the amputations below the level of the above-knee are the amputations through the distal femur and the transcondylar, supracondylar and Gritti–Stokes amputations.

The transcondylar amputation, in which the articular cartilage is removed in a procedure which is otherwise little different from the through-knee amputation, has little place in current practice. It has the disadvantage over through-knee amputation that the medullary cavity is opened.

All these operations divide the distal femur. In the transcondylar procedure this occurs at the level of the epicondyles and in the Gritti–Stokes procedure at the level of the adductor tubercle (but it is often higher in practice). In the supracondylar amputation the level of division should not be above the adductor tubercle.

The patellar tendon, quadriceps expansion and the capsule of the knee joint are divided anteriorly, whilst the biceps femoris, semitendinosus and semimembranosus are divided posteriorly with division of the heads of the gastrocnemius and plantaris. Medially, the gracilis and sartorius muscles are divided. The cruciate and collateral ligaments of the knee joint must be divided, together with the popliteal artery and vein behind the joint capsule. The sciatic nerve or medial and lateral popliteal components must be sectioned; bleeding from the companion artery may be a problem.

Where there is arterial occlusion this frequently involves the femoral and popliteal artery from the level of the adductor tendon. The distal branches of the cruciate anastomoses and the profunda femoris artery may carry the collateral circulation into the geniculate arteries which should be preserved to keep a circulation to the skin flaps. The blood supply to the end of a long bone is from the joint capsule and periosteum so that a minimum amount of periosteal elevation should be performed at the line of bone division.

These procedures provide a stump which acts as a long lever from the hip joint and most of the muscles are secured to the bone end giving the effect of a myodesis which preserves thigh muscle function.

All these amputations permit some end-bearing. In all but the transcondylar amputation the terminal area of the stump is small and part of the weight must be transmitted to the ischial tuberosity by the prosthesis. The stump is of cylindrical form and the tendency for the prosthesis to rotate must be controlled at hip

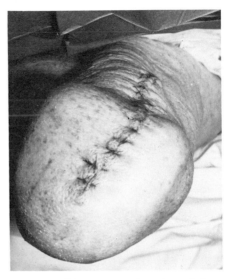

Fig. 12.4 The stump of a through-knee amputation with lateral flap (posterior view)

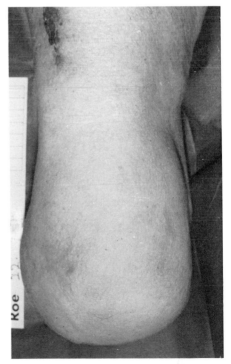

Fig. 12.5 The stump of a through-knee amputation with long anterior flap (anterior view)

level. The prosthesis for distal femoral amputations is therefore little different from that needed for a mid-thigh amputation. The proximity of the end of the stump to the level of the knee joint requires a knee mechanism outside the dimensions of the stump, which is no longer a prosthetic problem. It is not often realized that the line of weight transmission of a prosthesis for a Gritti–Stokes amputation falls behind the end of the stump, producing anteroposterior stresses on the thigh and necessitating a heavily built thigh corset.

These factors lead us to prefer a below- or through-knee amputation, but where a prosthesis is not likely to be worn the long lever of the supracondylar amputation is an advantage. This is especially so for the bilateral amputee who is thus able to roll over and move in bed, a feat which would be very difficult for the bilateral above-knee amputee.

Gritti–Stokes amputation

The patient is given a general anaesthetic and placed prone on the operating table. A tourniquet is not used in patients with vascular disease. A long anterior flap is formed based on the level of the femoral epicondyles, extending to the tibial tubercle, and a short posterior flap is cut not longer than 3 cm. The anterior flap is deepened down to the tibial periosteum and the knee-joint capsule and the patellar tendon is cleared from its insertion. This is easily performed with the knee flexed and further flexion allows the joint capsule to be opened wide to permit division of the cruciate and collateral ligaments. The semilunar cartilages are left attached to the tibial plateau. The posterior joint capsule is incised and the popliteal vessels exposed, ligated and divided. The medial and lateral popliteal nerves are divided and their arteries ligated.

The limb is extended to permit deepening of the posterior flap with division of the hamstring muscles and the heads of gastrocnemius, which allows the specimen to be removed. The joint capsule and the patella are retracted upwards and the femur is sawn across at the level of the adductor tubercle. The angle of the saw cut is crucial; this must be inclined by 10–15° to the transverse plane so that the tone of the extensor and flexor muscles will 'lock' it in place effectively. Previously, instability of the patella had been a problem — often a bar to limb-wearing by some of the patients.

The patella is best held in a large cotton pack while the articular surface is sawn off. The patella is drilled with a sharp bradawl to make four holes, and corresponding holes are drilled in the femoral cortex. This allows the patella to be firmly sutured to the end of the femur with braided nylon. The patella must be firmly fixed or bony union will not occur and a painful pseudo-arthrosis will result. The hamstring tendons are sutured to the patellar tendon to make a stable myodesis.

The skin and superficial fascia are closed with fine interrupted

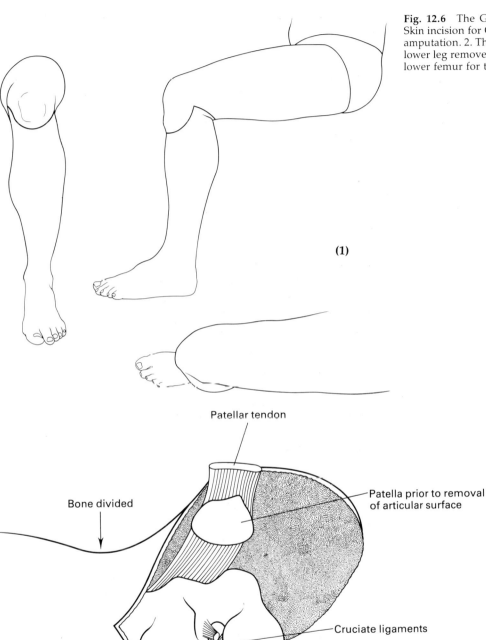

Fig. 12.6 The Gritti–Stokes amputation. 1. Skin incision for Gritti–Stokes supracondylar amputation. 2. The knee joint opened and the lower leg removed, allowing exposure of the lower femur for the supracondylar cut

(1)

Patellar tendon

Bone divided

Patella prior to removal of articular surface

Cruciate ligaments

Popliteal vein

Popliteal artery

Sciatic nerve

(2)

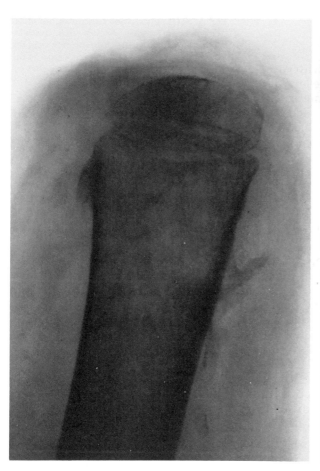

12.7

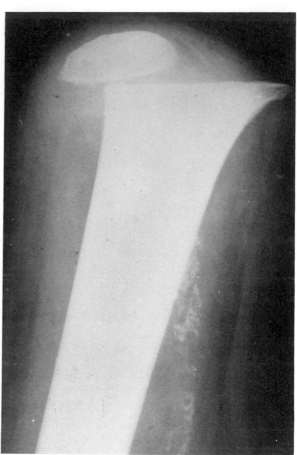

12.8

Fig. 12.7 A radiograph showing a successful classical Gritti–Stokes amputation

Fig. 12.8 A radiograph showing a displaced patella after a Gritti–Stokes amputation

nylon sutures and a suction tube drain is left in place for two days. The sutures are removed on the tenth day and the patient can use a pylon as soon as the wound is soundly healed. Walking with crutches is encouraged from the second postoperative day.

Two large series of patients treated by Gritti-Stokes amputation have shown that in the hands of a specialist team good results can be achieved by this technique. It is emphasized that the femoral remnant must not be too short, otherwise looseness of the patella will result; care must be taken over its absolute fixation. Recent developments in the prosthetic fitting of the Gritti–Stokes amputation have resulted in an improved limb with an acceptable knee-joint mechanism which has overcome many of the past prosthetic disadvantages. This consists of a total-contact socket combined with a conventional linkage knee-joint mechanism with modular assembly. The only disadvantage is the low axis of knee flexion, leading to prominence of the flexed knee and a short shin length.

Supracondylar amputation

The patient is given a general anaesthetic and placed prone on the operating table. A tourniquet is not used in patients with vascular disease. The skin flaps are semicircular based on the level of the femoral epicondyles with the knee flexed, and the anterior flap is cut down to the periosteum and joint capsule. The flaps are of equal length. The patellar tendon is detached from the tibial tubercle and the synovial cavity of the knee is opened, allowing the division of the cruciate and collateral ligaments of the knee joint. The semilunar cartilages are left attached to the tibial plateau. Acute flexion of the knee gives access to the cruciate ligaments.

The knee is then extended and the posterior flap cut through the superficial and deep fascia; the muscles are sectioned at the level of the skin incision and the vessels are carefully ligated. The sciatic nerve or its medial and lateral popliteal components are drawn down and the companion artery ligated before the ends retract.

The femur is divided with a Gigli saw above the condyles at the level of the adductor tubercle, taking care to make a horizontal cut which leaves a level flat end to the bone. The edges are filed to make a smooth end with slightly rounded corners. With the patella held in a towel clip the patellar tendon is peeled away by sharp dissection and the patella discarded. The anterior and posterior flaps are then approximated with thick catgut sutures so as to include the patellar tendon and quadriceps expansion in front and the hamstring tendons behind. A tube suction drain is placed close to the bone end and passed through the skin well above the wound. The skin is closed with fine interrupted nylon stitches without tension. Only a light dressing is required.

The drain is removed in 48 hours but the patient is kept in bed for five days. Thereafter, walking with crutches is encouraged and a pylon can be worn on the twelfth postoperative day.

Modified supracondylar amputation

This has been used at Roehampton, where the technique described above is followed, with the exception that the bone section is made as low as possible. The femur is drilled to allow the patellar and hamstring tendons to be sutured to the bone, which enables the medullary cavity of the femur to be closed and converts the amputation into an effective myodesis. The short equal flaps can be secured with Steristrips as there is no tension transmitted to the skin.

Prostheses for amputation through or near the knee joint

Amputation by disarticulation at the knee gives a stump which is fully end-bearing at knee level and which forms the longest

Fig. 12.9   The supracondylar amputation. 1.
The skin incision. 2. The femur divided at the
supracondylar level; the quadriceps expansion and hamstring muscles are divided ready
for attachment of the quadriceps to the hamstring tendon to form a myoplasty

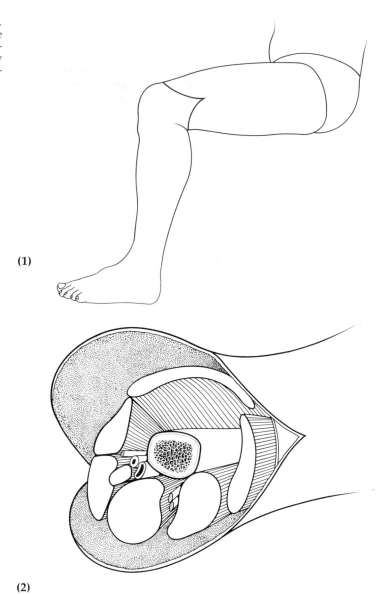

(1)

(2)

possible lever. It has little or no disturbance of its musculature, is
bulbous and rarely gives significant stump pain.

It is end-bearing and the level at which the patient has to
balance is at knee height and so balance is easier than in mid-
thigh amputations where the level of balance is at the proximal
end of the stump. The knee joint can be nearer the midline than
the centre of weight transmission, as in mid-thigh amputation, so
that the vertical load of the body has a shorter lever with which to
exert moment, while at the same time the counteracting forces
have a longer lever. Indeed, the inertia of body sway itself is
usually all that is required. There is then little or no pressure on

the distal lateral aspect of the stump nor in the groin.

This stump end-bearing must have full hip extension to have anteroposterior stability. The transfer of weight from the body to the prosthesis must be on a vertical line from the body's centre of gravity, passing in front of the artificial knee-joints and heel and behind the toe-break. With the long lever of the femur it requires only very little hip flexion to bring end-bearing in front of the foot, creating instability and rendering this amputation useless as an end-bearing stump. The forces other than weight transmission in both the stance and swing phase are similar to those in mid-thigh amputation. The length of the lever gives the best possible control of stability.

The bulbous nature of the stump is a prosthetic advantage for, as in the Syme's amputation, it is possible to use it to lift the prosthesis without any other suspension. There are other amputations at this level, for example the transcondylar and Gritti–Stokes, which some surgeons use for surgical reasons such as overcoming difficulties in healing. When these retain an end-bearing stump there is then a clinical purpose in doing them. However, some surgeons give as their reason the need to overcome the bulbous nature of the stump. It is emphasized that this bulbous property is one of the virtues of this amputation. Furthermore, in modifying the amputation there is always a reduction of the cross-section of the weight-bearing area. Simple transcondylar amputations will usually provide some end-bearing potential, although of less cross-section, and will retain the bulbous quality of the stump. Those amputations which re-position the patella under the femur increase the load six-fold on any unit area of skin. These stumps are rarely capable of taking full end-bearing and many cannot take any weight at the end at all. It is then necessary to exploit proximal bearing as in an above-knee amputation but without the benefit of the better mechanisms available for above-knee stumps of normal length. Hip flexion and stump pain are much commoner than in disarticulation at the knee and this operation is less favoured by the prosthetist for it combines many of the disadvantages of knee disarticulation on the above-knee prostheses, without their compensatory advantages.

Although the through-knee amputation may be fitted as a long above-knee stump using a metal or wood socket, or be fitted with a self-suspending leather lacing socket, the modern concept is to use a plastic socket and foam plastic liner in the same manner as a modern Syme's prosthesis.

An accurate cast is taken of the through-knee stump and on this is formed a plastic foam liner. The re-entrant areas on the outer surface of the liner are built up and then a hard socket made over the liner. The foam liner is split longitudinally to allow the bulbous end of the through-knee stump to enter the liner. When the stump and liner are pushed into the hard socket the liner is locked on the stump, suspending the limb securely. If necessary accessory suspension can be added.

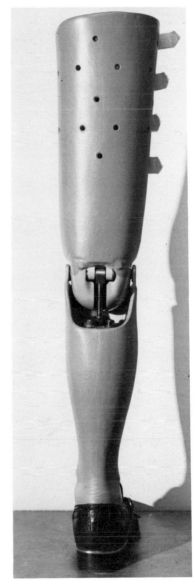

Fig. 12.10   A prosthesis for use after a Gritti–Stokes amputation

Fitted in this way the majority of through-knee stumps are fully end-bearing and no accessory suspension is required. The proximal socket trim-line can be left about 2.5 cm (1 in) below the ischial tuberosity. If the stump cannot accept full end-bearing the socket can be fashioned with an ischial-bearing brim fitting. The socket can be mounted on conventional side-steels and joints but the modern approach is to use a four-bar link knee unit and a tubular skin. This form of construction allows a one-piece soft cosmetic cover.

For geriatric amputees a hand-operated or semi-automatic knee lock should be provided.

13

Above-knee Amputations and Prostheses

Above-knee amputation is probably the most common in the lower limb and is frequently badly done. It is too often demoted to the end of the surgical list and delegated to the most junior and least experienced of the surgical staff. The operation, as still often performed, consists of little more than a guillotine amputation with only skin covering the bone end and often at an unnecessarily high level. Although such a procedure removes the pathology, a great deal is left to be desired in terms of comfort, rehabilitation and prosthetic management. The bone end is prominent, often with an adherent scar, and the skin is poorly nourished, cold and cyanotic. Retraction of muscles occurs leaving a conical stump which at one time satisfied prosthetic requirements by allowing a plug fit in a socket. This is a compromise far short of the ideal. The poorly covered bone often displaces laterally and is subject to excess pressure on the outer wall of the prosthesis, resulting in pain and occasionally in ulceration. The skin, because of its adherence to bone, is subject to excessive traction and pumping during walking and is prone to break down, producing painful fissures at the end of the stump. The unopposed action of the abductors and flexors produces a flexion–abduction contracture at the hip joint. This interferes considerably with the fitting of a prosthesis and grossly upsets the normal gait pattern. Such contractures are particularly associated with a short above-knee stump and they exaggerate the load and friction on the medial upper aspect of the thigh, producing painful callosities and implantation dermoids which frequently become infected. Limb wearing thus becomes difficult and sometimes impossible. Loss of length of the stump and muscle retraction results in diminished power.

This catalogue of criticisms of the standard above-knee amputation can be extended and it was this that prompted Dederich, Ertl, and others, dismayed by the appalling results of the above-knee amputations seen as the result of the Second World War, to advocate a different technique producing a more physiological stump, and it is this method which should be the standard practice today. Apart from the more obvious benefits of the myoplastic stump there is some evidence to support the view that phantom pain is a less frequent problem. It is postulated that some of the pain may be precipitated by venous stasis, anoxia and ischaemia, and that by producing a warm healthy stump with a good blood-flow many cases of phantom pain can be relieved.

As has been stressed elsewhere, to lose the knee joint is a grave disadvantage to any patient and above-knee amputations should

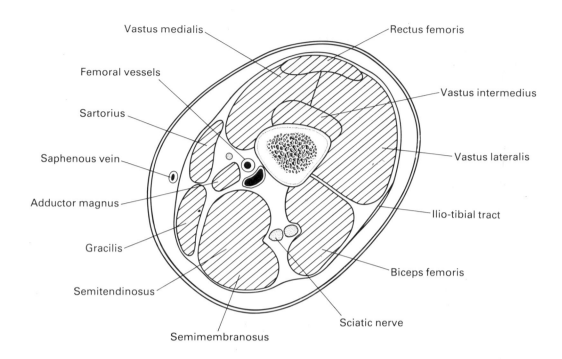

Fig. 13.1 Cross section of thigh at upper portion of lower third

not be performed where there is a possibility of an amputation at a lower level being successful. In malignant disease there may be no choice but in trauma, infection, and particularly ischaemic disease every effort should be made to retain the knee.

MID-THIGH AMPUTATION

Technique

General anaesthesia is desirable and a tourniquet is used except in ischaemic disease. The proximity to the rectum is responsible for the occasional infection with anaerobic organisms. Metronidazole suppositories and cotton-wool cover for the perineum will reduce this possibility. The patient is placed supine with a sandbag under the buttock. From the point of view of prosthetic management the longer the stump (within certain limits) the better. The main limiting factor is the room required in the prosthesis for the knee mechanism. This is approximately 11 cm, so that bone section is about 13 cm above knee-joint line. Equal anterior and posterior skin flaps are fashioned so that the scar will be terminal. They should be cut long at first and squared off to produce a blunt-nosed stump. They may be trimmed at the end of the operation. The incisions begin medially and laterally opposite the proposed site of bone section. The skin is dissected off, with subcutaneous tissue and deep fascia as one layer.

The muscles should be separated into four basic groups. The

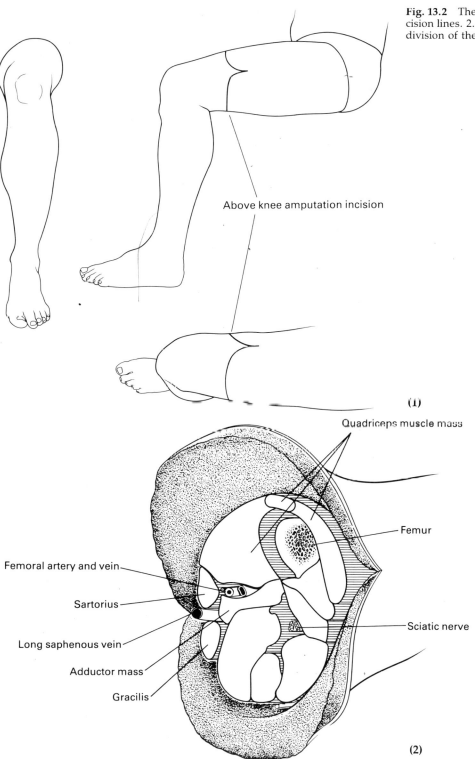

Fig. 13.2   The above-knee amputation. 1. Incision lines. 2. The completed dissection and division of the femur

Above knee amputation incision

(1)

Quadriceps muscle mass

Femur

Femoral artery and vein

Sartorius

Sciatic nerve

Long saphenous vein

Adductor mass

Gracilis

(2)

extensors and the flexors of the knee are obvious and easily defined. The adductors at the proposed level of section are a good deal smaller and the abductors consist basically of the iliotibial tract. Marker stitches are placed in these four muscle groups at the proposed level of bone section, in order that they may be sutured together at the correct physiological tension after amputation. These four muscle bundles are sectioned distally and dissected just proximal to the level of bone section as four basic groups spaciously orientated rather than anatomically determined. The femoral vessels are displayed and dissected to as high a level as is conveniently possible and divided. The femoral vein and artery are separately doubly ligated. The sciatic nerve is gently pulled down and cleanly divided so that it withdraws out of the wound. There is often considerable initial haemorrhage from the vessel that accompanies the sciatic nerve so the nerve can be ligated with fine catgut if the vessel itself cannot be secured, but usually this is not required.

Numerous methods have been advocated in the past to prevent neuroma formation. These have included ligation, cauterization, injection with phenol or other chemicals, and even implantation into muscle and bone, but they have generally been unsuccessful. Neuroma formation is inevitable and care must be taken that it occurs in areas free from possible adherence to tissues in the stump and not exposed to pressure in a prosthesis, as pain is then almost inevitable.

The femoral shaft is cleared to a level 5 cm below the proposed level of section. A circular incision is made in the periosteum and this structure is carefully stripped up proximally as a sheath. In the young this is easy as the periosteum is a substantial structure, but in the elderly it becomes very thin and tenuous. The bone is divided with an amputation saw or cantilever power saw and the bone edges are carefully filed to produce a smooth surface. The periosteal cuff is sutured over the open medullary cavity, effectively sealing it. This helps to maintain a normal intramedullary circulation, which may have some beneficial effect on the metabolism of the femoral shaft and will prevent the establishment of arteriovenous shunts.

A more normal pattern of blood flow is thus established in the stump and the possibility of local anoxia and pain is diminished. At this stage the tourniquet is released and haemostasis is secured. The groups of muscles are now sutured over the bone end at the normal resting tension, the stay-sutures acting as guides. Abductors and adductors are sutured first, with care being taken to place sutures above and below the femoral stump so that it is completely sheathed in muscle and cannot escape. Many surgeons advocate drilling the bone end to enable strong catgut sutures to anchor the muscle groups and prevent displacement of the bone end. Sutures should also anchor the muscle layer to the periosteum covering the bone end. There is a risk otherwise that the muscles will remain free as a sling over the end of the bone and produce a bursa deep to them which may be painful. The

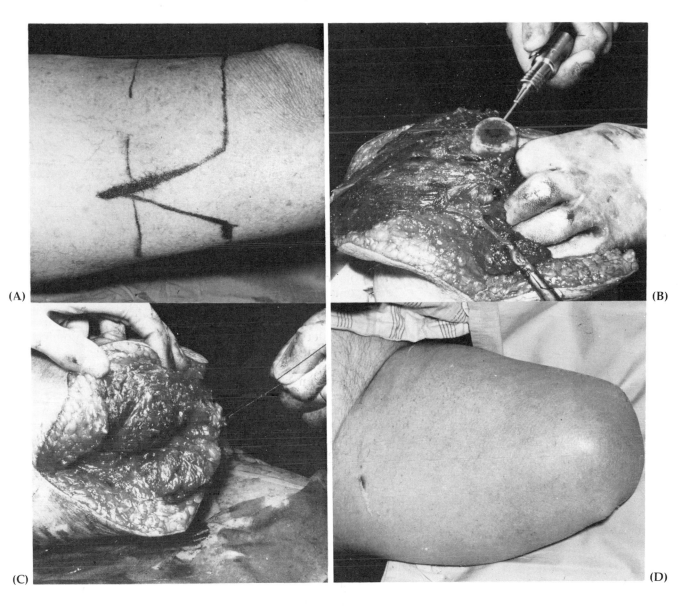

(A)

(B)

(C)

(D)

extensors and the flexors are then sutured after trimming to the required length. An alternative technique, described by Professor Murdoch, is to cut the hamstrings, the hip adductors and abductors flush with the end of the femoral shaft and to anchor them there by sutures passed through drill-holes through the lower end of the femoral shaft. The quadriceps tendon is then sutured over the cut femoral shaft and to the hamstrings posteriorly. Fascia should be sutured as a separate layer. The subcutaneous tissue should be sutured separately if bulky and the skin closed by interrupted sutures. Suction drainage should always be used. The suture line is dressed and sealed with plastic

Fig. 13.3 The above-knee amputation in progress. A, Preoperative marking of skin flaps and bone sections. B, Drilling the holes. C, Suturing the muscle groups. D, The final stump

spray, the wound and thigh covered with wool and a light plaster cast applied. This is more effective than a crêpe bandage in controlling terminal swelling and is more comfortable. The sutures are retained for 14 days. An active programme of exercise begun preoperatively is continued postoperatively and pursued vigorously. Pylon-walking may be started as soon as the wound is healed.

The mid-thigh prosthesis and its biomechanics

In the United Kingdom it has been traditional to distinguish between long mid-thigh stumps, in which the control of the prosthesis is by the stump alone, and short stumps, which require a metal hip joint to give additional stability. There is a difference between using and not using a metal hip joint but it is related more to the mental and physical abilities of the patient and the amputation surgery than to the actual length of the stump.

These amputations through the shaft of the femur are proximal-bearing. The basic artificial knee joint is a spindle running transversely below the stump on which the shin (shank) moves. This spindle is placed at the level of the mean anatomical knee axis, approximately 3 cm above the knee joint level and, for stability, behind the vertical line of the body's centre of gravity and the ankle joint. The amputation stump must therefore have a bone section shorter than this and allow for soft tissue. Any amputation within 6 cm of the knee joint, whether it is end-bearing or not, will have to have the type of prosthesis used for knee disarticulation and its variants. Even with bone section at 6 cm above the knee joint the surgeon is doing his patient a disservice: only a simple axis can be supplied, and currently available knee mechanisms giving improved stability and alignment in the stance phase and control of the swing phase cannot be included. To utilize the best of the controls and sockets available will require a bone section 14 cm above the knee joint in the United Kingdom and 10 cm in North America. At the present time there are restrictions imposed on the surgeon by prosthetic considerations but new methods of making sockets and new knee mechanisms are being investigated, which should eventually remove this constraint.

At the other extreme we have to consider how short a stump may be. The shortest stump which can be useful to a patient will depend on his physique and mentality. The physical contours, bulk and firmness of the tissues are also important factors. Taking these factors into account the shortest useful stump is four fingerbreadths (8 cm) below the pubic ramus. The prostheses described are for amputations through the shaft of the femur between these two levels.

Sockets for mid-thigh prostheses

The sockets of these prostheses are traditionally proximal-bearing and are ischial-bearing at the present time, although with new surgical and prosthetic techniques an element of more distal loading is now common. There are a number of different types of socket at present in use. The shape of the socket has to accommodate the tendon of adductor longus at its origin, the ischial tuberosity and the great trochanter. The soft tissues may be distorted to some extent to meet the mechanical requirements of the socket provided the total circumference is adequate. The types of socket include the conventional or plug fit socket, the 'H' socket and the quadrilateral socket. There may or may not be total contact to the surface of the stump. The socket may be suction/self-suspending or may require the addition of an external suspension system.

The conventional or plug fit socket

This socket was in use for centuries until the end of the Second World War. Many wore it in comfort for years when properly fitted and, indeed, it is in satisfactory use by some patients at the present day. The body's weight is in part transmitted by the glutei and ischial tuberosity but also to a large extent by circumferential pressure round the whole of the proximal stump. Properly made, these sockets were somewhat triangular, encompassing the ischial tuberosity and great trochanter but they are now more often made with a circular cross section. The posterior rim of the socket is rolled out to provide a seating and runs obliquely downward to the medial wall. The anterior wall is at the same height as the posterior wall and runs obliquely upwards, following a line above 3 cm below the inguinal fold to the trochanter. There was no end-bearing in these sockets and the terminal one-third of the stump was rarely in contact with the socket except laterally during the stance phase.

These sockets are still used for patients who have long been accustomed to them and who have no difficulties arising from their use. The grossly obese whose ischial tuberosity cannot be located may be better with this type of socket. Conversely, the very thin elderly patient with lax skin and a small, poorly covered ischial tuberosity may not tolerate ischial seating and may be better with the conventional socket. Lastly, the patient with the very short bulky abducting stump may need this socket in order to remain in his socket when sitting and to maintain control of the prosthesis in the swing phase of walking.

The socket has, however, been a source of discomfort for a large number, possibly the majority, of its wearers. Indeed, many who protest that they are comfortable using this socket will show clear evidence of chronic trauma to the skin and soft tissues on the medial side of the thigh in the groin. If persuaded to use a modern socket they will admit that they had previously put up

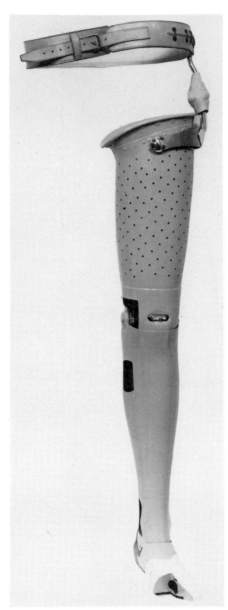

Fig. 13.4 A conventional above-knee prosthesis with pelvic band

with much discomfort. Because the socket is a trumpet-shaped cone, with the rim running obliquely, the stump sinks into it until it can go no further. The weight is largely borne by the soft tissue on the medial side of the thigh and over the adductor tendon because of the obliquity of the rim, as well as the need to produce pressure proximally on the medial wall for stability in the stance phase. The pistoning of the stump within the socket produces friction in this area and milks a roll of fat over the medial rim of the socket giving rise to sebaceous or epidermoid cysts.

'H' and 'quadilateral' sockets

It was the prevalence of cysts which led to the development of the 'H' socket and the 'quadrilateral' socket. There are sometimes heated arguments between the protagonists of each socket, but basic conception and biomechanics of each are similar. The 'H' socket is the one most commonly used in the United Kingdom, the quadrilateral socket being more common in North America and continental Europe, though there are some variations of techique. Correctly made sockets of either type can be used successfully by patients.

Both sockets depend on a level shelf as a seating for the ischial tuberosity. It is sometimes suggested that this seating takes the whole body-weight. Since at most only 3–4 cm^2 under the ischial tuberosity can be load-bearing, it is manifest that the load would be unacceptable if all the weight were taken on the ischial tuberosity. It does, however, provide a lug which prevents the stump being driven into the socket at heel contact, thus preventing an impact on the adductor tendon. It is a major area of load-bearing but the posterior rim of the socket also distributes weight on the buttock and some weight at low pressure is taken circumferentially. The anterior walls of both sockets are kept high to hold the stump back on to the ischial tuberosity. In the 'H' socket, room is given to the adductor tendon and the medial wall then passes posteromedially so that a triangular flange provides a seating under the ischial tuberosity. It then curves posteriorly and laterally to give room for the gluteus maximus tendon, and passes anteriorly, curving upwards and in behind the trochanter, and then out to give room for this bony structure. Passing under the anterior superior iliac spine it is flattened to give counterpressure obliquely backwards and medially so as to hold the stump on to the tuber seating, and then descends medially to the adductor region.

In the quadrilateral socket the medial wall runs posteriorly from the adductor region until it reaches a level when a right-angle turn will bring the posterior wall under the ischial tuberosity. It then passes laterally with less allowance for the glutei and without curving in behind the trochanter. It is not flattened under the anterior superior spine but is curved to give a bulge over the femoral triangle, and this gives a posteriorly directed counterpressure to hold the stump on to the ischial seating. In both sockets it should be noted that there is room for the adductor tendon and the great trochanter and that the ischial tuberosity is firmly ensconced on a levelled seating. In both sockets the lateral wall of the socket should be fashioned to provide lateral support to within 3 cm of the cut end of the femur so as to provide a lever for the abductors to work on.

These sockets can be made of wood or metal. The quadrilateral brim shape has lent itself for use as a jig to mould the proximal part of the plaster cast of the stump for making a socket out of plastic. These sockets were originally intended to be open-ended. While the transfer of weight to the socket is still proximal it is now considered that the soft tissues should be supported terminally. Sockets are now total-contact sockets unless the end of the stump is so unhealthy that end contact cannot be tolerated. If wood or metal sockets are used, sponge rubber or Silastic foam injections are made to give this terminal contact. Plastic sockets made to a cast of the stump may themselves provide the end support without padding.

The total surface bearing socket

In the United Kingdom a socket has been developed which is not ischial-bearing. The original suggestion was made by Inman of California that the body weight might be transmitted evenly through the soft tissues in such a way that the whole stump contributes to support. Such a socket has now been provided in the United Kingdom. Its use is at present limited to those who suspend their limbs by suction or muscular contraction.

Earlier efforts to produce these sockets involved making a cast with the patient standing and putting weight on to the stump during casting. This tended to push the soft tissue upwards, increasing the tranverse diameter, and to force the femoral remnant downwards. As the limb was lifted the femur rose inside the soft tissues and the stump elongated so that its circumference lessened.

The present sockets are made by compressing the soft tissues with specially woven elastic material to the calculated pressure of about 45 kPa needed to support the body while at the same time stressing them distally, so that the femoral remnant is withdrawn as far as it can be within the soft tissues. A cast is then taken from which a plastic socket is made. When the patient wears the socket the stump is pulled into it so that it completely fills the socket. It is then in the shape required to transmit the load evenly at the calculated unit loading when standing, and when the limb is lifted it responds immediately because the femur cannot rise further within the soft tissues. This socket has not yet received acceptance in North America but is being increasingly used in the United Kingdom and some European countries, and is known as the total surface bearing socket.

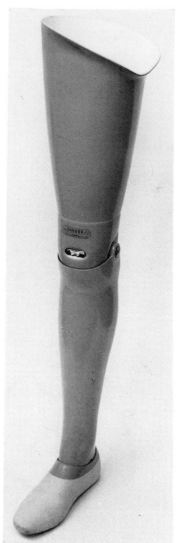

Fig. 13.5 An above-knee prosthesis with a suction valve

Socket alignment

So far only the transmission of the body's weight to the socket has been discussed and not the alignment of the socket, nor the other forces which are present between the socket and the stump. With amputations through the shaft of the femur there is a need to set up the socket in some 5–10° flexion, even if there is no flexion deformity of the hip. This is necessary firstly because there is a slight apparent flexion deformity due to the normal anterior bowing of the femur and, secondly, because extension of the hip is limited by the Y-shaped iliofemoral ligament. In using an artificial limb, about 5° of extension beyond the vertical is required if excessive pressure is not to occur anteriorly on the cut end of the femur. There is also some degree of muscular imbalance due to amputation, however well it may be done, for there is a greater loss of hip extensors than flexors. In the elderly there is also a tendency for the stump to be in some flexion when relaxed even if full active extension is possible. Patients with degenerative changes in their lumbar spines may then complain of backache which can often be relieved by increasing the flexion of the socket in the prosthesis. There are also patients who have a flexion contracture of the hip before amputation or who develop one afterwards. The socket must then be set up in flexion to accommodate this deformity plus the 5–10° to allow extension of the artificial limb. If extreme, such socket flexion will limit the stride, for when the prosthesis is vertical the stump is in flexion.

While maximum load is usually considered to be on the ischial seating the centre of the load is anterior to this and is usually considered to be at the mid-trochanter level. Indeed, if all the weight were transmitted to the posterior rim of the socket it would produce prosthetic difficulties, for to be stable the artificial knee joint needs to be posterior to a vertical line from the point of loading.

In static alignment the socket must be placed into its container in the necessary flexion so that the weight is transmitted in front of the knee joint. Insufficient flexion will cause the patient to lean forward and may give rise to painful pressure on the cut end of femur. Too much flexion will shorten the stride when walking and also give an unnecessarily unsightly bulge to the prosthesis.

The socket also needs to be set with the lateral wall in appreciable adduction. There is a tendency for the stump to abduct, particularly in the higher levels of mid-thigh amputation, because there is a greater loss of adductor muscle than abductor muscle. It is necessary to give stability in standing by pressures down the lateral aspect of the femur to prevent pelvic rotation due to the body's weight being medial to the socket. If the socket is abducted it is difficult to stabilize the hip and more of the pressure is distributed towards the distal end of the femur which is already subject to some pressure. The shorter the femoral stump the greater this distal pressure is, as the effective lever about which the lateral force operates is lessened. Indeed, in a short stump it is not mechanically possible to contract the hip abductors strongly enough to prevent a Trendelenburg gait. It is then necessary to introduce an additional lever system by using a stick (cane) in the opposite hand. It is important to know this, for some patients with short stumps may become discouraged because unless they use a stick (cane) they are unable to walk without a limp.

The other force required to balance the body weight is compounded of the inertia of the body sway and proximal pressure on the medial wall of the socket. The latter can be relieved in some types of suspension by pressure on the opposite pelvic wall.

In walking during the stance phase there is a changing pattern from heel-strike to toe-off. At heel-strike the foot attempts to plantar flex causing the shin to tend to rotate forward and the knee to flex. To prevent this, when simple knee mechanisms are in use, the thigh stump has to be extended. This gives rise to high pressures on the lower part of the back of the stump and on the upper rim anteriorly. The latter is partly due to the mechanical effect of the artificial limb trying to rotate, as well as the strong contractions of the hip extensors thrusting the stump forward in the socket. This pattern has to continue until the artificial limb reaches the vertical and gains its inherent stability, unless a stabilizing device to lock the knee is incorporated.

The pattern of forces acting on the stump then changes to be reversed at toe-off, the stump thrusting forward in the socket to flex the knee and swing the leg forward. In patients using a free knee this thrust is vigorous so as to make the knee joint flex passively and raise the foot off the ground. At the end of the swing phase, the hip extensors again come into play to decelerate the prosthesis and cause the shin (shank) to swing into extension.

Suspension for the prostheses

The suspension used with these prostheses may be divided into two major groups:
1   Those with hip stability in which the stump must control the prosthesis. These can be further subdivided into suction and non-suction sockets.
2   Those with hip instability in which a metal hip joint assists in controlling the prosthesis.

Suction sockets are often spoken of as if they were intrinsically different from other sockets but they are not. Suction is a method of suspension and at the present time is misnamed. It has long been thought that if a partial vacuum could be created below the stump it would suspend the artificial limb. Many years ago this was attempted with the conventional plug fit socket with almost uniformly disastrous results, for the suction pulled the stump further and further into the socket, increasing the circumferential pressure and producing the effects of 'dry cupping' of a bygone age. Suction was then abandoned until the introduction of the

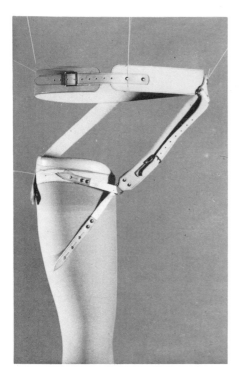

Fig. 13.6   A modified version of a silesian belt

ischial seating sockets. With these the stump was no longer sucked into the socket. Terminal congestion was the rule and only a limited number of patients could wear them. Even those who could wear these sockets successfully for a time would suddenly develop terminal congestion after some years. There were considerable arguments about the size of the chamber required below the stump and the negative pressure desirable. Special valves were designed, varying from simple bungs to valves allowing expulsion of air as the stump pistoned down. In the United Kingdom a valve was used which allowed not only the expulsion of air but also its admission when the negative pressure exceeded a predetermined level. Eventually it was found that the terminal congestion in this socket and in others could be overcome by support of the terminal soft tissues. Indeed, the enemy of the suction socket is suction. These sockets are now total-contact sockets.

During the stance phase there is a positive pressure within the socket. In the swing phase the pressures are equal only to the weight of the prosthesis distributed over the surface of the stump, because the close fit prevents air entering. The patient introduces the stump into the socket by pulling it in with a stocking or a bandage, so that the whole of the socket is filled.

To use this type of socket the patient needs to maintain a constant stump volume. Quite small losses of weight will cause the socket to be too loose so that the limb falls off, whereas any added weight will make it too tight. The patient also needs the mentality and physical abilities to control the prosthesis with the stump alone and the stump itself must not be too ill-fashioned. There are many patients whose weight fluctuates but who meet these other criteria. For them the limb can be suspended by some non-rigid material to the waist or over the shoulders. There are many variations of this suspension and the following is only a brief outline of some of them.

1   *'Silesian' belt*. This is a simple belt originally used in Germany to give added suspension and provide peace of mind in suction socket wearers. A stud is fixed to the lateral rim of the socket which is kept sufficiently high and to which is attached a belt that passes behind the body, round the pelvis and then attaches at a lower level to the front of the socket. It is useful in suction socket wearers with short stumps, not so much as a supplement to the suction but as a counterpressure to relieve the pressure on the medial side of the stump in the stance phase. It is also sometimes the only suspension needed by active patients with muscular stumps who for other reasons cannot use a suction socket. There are now variations of the silesian belt that provide more positive suspension that the original design. An example of a modified version of a silesian belt is shown in Fig. 13.6.

2   *Waist belt*. Provided the patient has a waist the limb can be suspended by leather straps, often crossing in front of and behind the socket; by roller cords running through housed rollers on the medial and lateral aspects of the thigh; or by wide elastics at the front and back. These latter two suspensions are widely used by women. When abdominal operations or obesity prevent the use of a waist belt, a shoulder suspension or similar device may be used.

3 *Suspension with hip stability and metal hip joint.* The young patient with the short stump, patients with paralysis, and the enfeebled elderly may not be able to control a prosthesis by use of the stump alone and will need the addition of a metal hip joint and pelvic band. To give the greatest possible stability a uniaxial joint is placed lateral to the hip joint, its lower member being attached to the top of the lateral wall of the socket and the upper steel to a metal band which runs forward and backwards for about 15 cm within the waist belt. This band is intended to run under the iliac crest and to be held firmly against the wall of the pelvis to give firm support. Few patients use the rigid pelvic band in this way, largely because it then lives up to its name. The waist belt is commonly left a little loose or the prosthetist is persuaded to lengthen the upper steel so that it becomes a waist rather than a pelvic belt, both giving laxity in the fixation.

This laxity is, however, often necessary because when the pelvic band is firmly held on to the pelvis the lateral sway of the body either rips the lower steels out of the socket or snaps the upper steel. The rotations of the pelvis also raise torques in the system, leading to failure. For this reason the pelvic band is sometimes hinged. This allows some compliance to the pelvic rotation and also to the changing abdominal contours of the corpulent as they sit. Some of the lateral sway can be accommodated by introducing a joint with limited lateral movement into the upper steel. These modifications do, however, reduce the stability provided by the system and if used successfully may indicate that one of the other forms of suspension might be appropriate.

Also in common use, particularly in the United Kingdom, are the so-called double swivel pelvic bands which were originally designed to give freedom of suspension without limiting movement. The steel joining the hip joint to the pelvic band is attached to it by a joint allowing rotation in a vertical axis. The hip joint is then attached to the prosthesis through a horizontal stirrup attached at the front and back to give a horizontal axis running anteroposteriorly.

These hip joints are not now so widely used as there is an increasing use of either non-metallic waist belts or suction suspension for patients who previously might have used them. The use of a modified silesian belt has also helped to replace the double swivel set up.

Foot and ankle mechanisms

These mechanisms are the same as for lower levels of amputation. The artificial limb is a long lever and minor errors of angulation at foot level are exaggerated at the hip level and vice versa. If there is too much dorsiflexion of the foot the patient will have to extend the hip to put the whole sole of the foot in contact with the ground or he will have to stand on the heel only, which is an unstable position with a tendency to knee-shoot. The latter is sometimes utilized by the active when walking, as it allows them speedy movement into toe-off. This preference is commonly an indication that the limb has been set up with too much alignment stability (the knee axis being too far behind the load line), which makes it difficult to flex the knee at the end of the stance phase. In the elderly, or for anyone in a standing occupation, the need to maintain extension of the hip for stabilization is tiring.

Conversely, if the foot is set in excessive plantar flexion it throws the prosthesis backwards, so that the patient feels he is falling backwards when standing and will have to bend at the hips to bring his centre of gravity over the foot. It also makes it difficult to initiate the step and the patient will complain that it feels like walking uphill.

Knee mechanisms

The knee mechanism may be divided into two groups: those concerned with stance-phase control and those concerned with swing-phase control.

Stance-phase controls

Semi-automatic lock. This is the simplest and lightest of these controls. The artificial knee automatically locks with full extension when the patient stands up and remains locked until positively released for sitting down. It is suitable for the feeble, particularly the elderly, but may be required by those who, because of paralysis or a very short stump, cannot control the prosthesis with the stump even when maximum alignment stability has been provided.

Hand-operated lock. This lock is applied voluntarily by the patient to the knee joint. It is usually combined with swing-phase controls and in itself it is not heavy. It is suitable for patients who wish to walk with a freely swinging knee but whose occupation or environment requires stability. Going down slopes or walking on a factory floor, where unexpected unevenness might cause the patient to fall in dangerous surroundings, will make it necessary to provide some locking device for all but those with strong stumps and quick reactions. They are now becoming largely obsolete with the introduction of modern stabilizing knee systems.

Stabilizing knee joints. The semi-automatic lock and the hand-operated lock act at all phases of the gait pattern. The hand-operated lock functions only when it is applied. They both operate to the detriment of the swing phase when applied and the hand-operated lock only provides stability during the stance phase if the patient anticipates its need. Knee joints are now available which allow free movement of the knee in the swing phase but effectively lock the knee up to 30° flexion during the stance phase. There are three main groups, hydraulic, friction, and polycentric.

1 *Hydraulic stabilizing knees.* These are usually combined with a hydraulic swing-phase mechanism in which a piston forces a fluid through an orifice. To provide a locking mechanism basically requires that as weight is transmitted to the knee joint the orifice is closed, thereby preventing further movement of the piston and locking the knee joint at that position. This is an over-simplification of what are most complex engineering designs but all such devices work basically on this principle.

2 *Friction stabilizing knees.* There are a number of these now available, two being in current use in the United Kingdom. In these systems the principle is that when a load is applied to the knee the thigh displaces slightly towards the shin, thereby bringing two braking surfaces into contact and preventing further movement. When the load is removed springs separate the surfaces, allowing free movement of the knee once again. These systems are effective in holding the full weight of the body in 30° flexion. They add weight to the prosthesis and therefore may absorb more energy in movement but this is probably more than compensated for by the reduction in muscular and nervous energy required to maintain the knee in extension with a simple knee joint

   (a) *Bouncy knee lock.* This device is a resilient flexion resistor built into friction knee stabilizer that allows a limited amount of knee flexion to take place when the prosthesis is in the stance phase of the gait cycle, thus simulating the action of the knee. An example of such a device is the Bouncy knee/Blatchford stabilized knee unit.

4 *Polycentric knee joints.* Polycentric knee joints, usually in the form of four-bar linkages of various geometry, have been introduced from time to time for many years. The designs all seek to facilitate the maintenance of knee extension during the stance phase by using the geometry to manipulate the path of the instantaneous axis of knee flexion to advantage. None has yet had wide acceptance, at least in the United Kingdom.

Swing-phase controls

During the swing phase of walking with the prosthesis it is necessary to modify its movement. These modifications are accelerators and decelerators acting on the various parts of the prosthesis at different phases of the swing.

The swing will however be modified by a change of the total mass of the prosthesis and its distribution relative to the prosthetic joints. The benefit conferred by a heavy mechanism may in fact be due to its weight providing a better pendular characteristic to the prosthesis, rather than any action it may have. Conversely, the weight of a mechanism may so adversely affect the gait as to negate its beneficial action. The addition therefore of ankle and foot mechanisms which add weight distally, thereby lengthening the pendulum, will be a disadvantage. Stance-phase knee controls which are incorporated with the shin (shank) will affect the swing in different way from stance-phase controls of similar weight incorporated into the thigh member. Both will affect the swing of the prosthesis and are therefore to this extent swing-phase controls. Similarly semi-automatic or hand-operated knee locks affect the swing of the prosthesis by preventing flexion of the knee and convert the prosthesis from a compound pendulum to a simple pendulum. The effect therefore of stance-phase controls upon the swing phase must be considered when prescribing the limb.

The acceleration and deceleration mechanisms added to the prosthesis specifically to modify the movements during the swing are referred to as swing-phase controls. The accelerators are springs or rubbers which are either compressed or stretched to rebound. In the knee this can be a spring operating on a lever running into the calf (the internal calf spring) or an elastic pick-up (kick strap) attached to the top of the shin (shank) and either the top of the socket or the waist belt. As the thigh thrusts forwards in the socket the inertia of the shin (shank) causes it to lag behind thus flexing the knee and causing the foot to rise off the ground. The calf spring or the pick-up (kick strap) is then stretched, at which time it acts as a decelerator and rebounds to accelerate the shin (shank) forward. If the pick-up (kick strap) also is attached to the waist belt it will act about the hip joint to assist in the movement of the thigh piece.

The decelerations are required at the extremes of the swing phase, operating on flexion after toe-off and on extension before heel contact. The decelerator in earlier limbs was the inherent friction in leather bushes in the knee joint. The inherent friction of the earlier knee joints also had a mechanical stop which prevented hyperextension of the knee by completing deceleration of the shin at heel contact. This mechanical stop is still used routinely.

Modern bearings have less friction. If left unmodified the heel rises higher and higher the faster the patient walks and the knee may still be flexed when heel contact should be taking place. If there is no deceleration before full extension the shank jerks the whole leg forward as it comes on to the mechanical stops at full extension. Dampers must therefore be introduced. In the United Kingdom the common simple friction device consists of a brake drum fixed to the knee spindle and therefore fixed relative to the shin. A band lined with brake material and fixed relative to the thigh is applied to the periphery of the drum. This can be adjusted to vary the amount of friction suitable for a given walking speed but in use it cannot adjust itself to changes of walking pace. Similar devices are in common use throughout the world. This device will prevent excessive heel rise and decelerate the shin at the end of the swing phase, but it also operates throughout the swing phase causing purposeless and wasteful energy expenditure. There are also, however, mechanical systems employing multivane disc-braking devices which only operate at the extremes of the swing phase and are similarly not self-adjusting to walking speed.

For many years now various hydraulic swing-phase controls have been widely used in North America and elsewhere, although constant-friction controls have been also used. Their benefit may in part have been due to their weight characteristics, for patients have been known to prefer them even when all the oil has escaped and the mechanism is not functioning. The disadvantages of these mechanisms are, firstly, that they are weighty with the weight in the shin and, secondly, that they are not leak-proof, with mechanical as well as social disadvantages. Most of them require frequent maintenance. Their particular advantage is that they can be designed to be immediately adaptive to changes in walking speed. Pneumatic swing-phase controls are now available which are lighter and do not soil clothing if they leak.

Both these systems depend upon the rate at which fluid — whether liquid or gas — can be forced through an orifice by a piston acting in a cylinder. They can be arranged so that there is no resistance in the middle of the swing and so that they only come into play at the extremes of the swing phase. The pneumatic devices are automatically self-adjusting to the speed of walking but less completely so than hydraulic systems.

Prosthetic prescribing

In prescribing the type of socket suspension and mechanism, the surgeon and prosthetists have a wide range of possibilities. They must take into account the patient's mental and physical abilities, the length, configuration and power of his amputation stump, his occupational and recreational demands and his environment.

Elderly, feeble patients with other disease conditions will need only a limited use within the environment of the house. For them functional stability to reduce effort and remove fear is the main requirement. They need a rigid pelvic band and semi-automatic knee lock in the lightest possible limb. The young active man with a good stump needs suction suspension without any added hip stability in the stance phase. For him swing-phase controls give the nearest possible approach to a normal gait, for which weight is a minor consideration. Between these extremes are all types of patient with varying conditions and occupations who may need stability at the hip joint or knee or both. Will the stabilizing knee joint be adequate or should there be a more positive lock? Is the added weight of a swing-phase control needed by the patient whose pull is limited by other disease? What is the likelihood of deterioration in the patient? Whereas the young man with a life expectancy of years needs the most mobility he can manage, the old man needs stability before mobility. It may be better to initiate him in a prosthesis he can manage within two to three years, by which time his physical condition has deteriorated, rather than give him a complex mechanism within his present capabilities.

14

Hindquarter Amputations and Prostheses

DISARTICULATION OF THE HIP

This is an amputation of the lower limb below the pelvic girdle in which the femur is detached at the hip joint. All the muscles controlling the lower limb are severed at the time of amputation, leaving no projection capable of any lever function, but in contrast to a hindquarter amputation the stable bony pelvis remains which is capable of weight-bearing on the ischial tuberosity and pelvic wall. The pubic ramus, the iliac crest and a close-fitting rigid socket enclosing the whole pelvis can be moved with precision. The powerful accurate movements which result can swing the prosthetic limb, although acting at a very poor mechanical advantage.

Hip disarticulation entails division of all the structures passing from the pelvis into the lower limb and all those attached to the outside of the bony hemipelvis. The sciatic, obturator and femoral nerves are all sectioned. The femoral vessels are the largest to be divided but the branches of the obturator, superior and inferior gluteal arteries must be identified and secured. The anterior muscles which must be divided are the pectineus, psoas major, sartorius, tensor fascia lata and the rectus femoris and

Fig. 14.1 The structures encountered during disarticulation at the hip

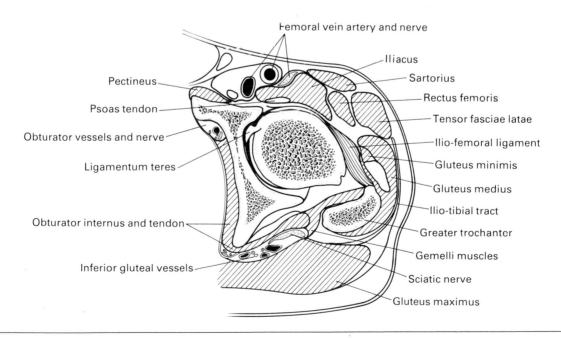

Femoral vein artery and nerve

Iliacus

Pectineus

Sartorius

Psoas tendon

Rectus femoris

Obturator vessels and nerve

Tensor fasciae latae

Ligamentum teres

Ilio-femoral ligament

Gluteus minimis

Gluteus medius

Ilio-tibial tract

Obturator internus and tendon

Greater trochanter

Gemelli muscles

Inferior gluteal vessels

Sciatic nerve

Gluteus maximus

Fig. 14.2   The stump of a hip disarticulation

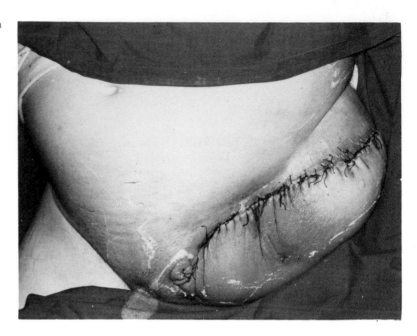

medially the gracilis, adductor longus, adductor magnus and adductor brevis.

Posteriorly the hamstrings from the ischial tuberosity, the semimembranosus, the semitendonosus and the biceps femoris are divided. The posterior incision will divide the gluteus maximus, gluteus medius and gluteus minimus together with the piriformis, obturator internus and the superior and inferior gemelii. Obturator externus and quadratus femoris will also be divided. The capsule of the hip joint is opened and completely divided, cutting the ligamentum teres to permit external rotation and dislocation of the head of the femur.

Technique

As large muscle masses must be divided, a hypotensive anaesthetic technique and the use of surgical diathermy is recommended. The patient lies flat with the hip raised by a large sandbag under the sacrum and an assistant must be available to control the leg.

Although racquet incisions are described, the long posterior flap of Kelly is preferred. The anterior incision extends from the adductor longus tendon to just above the greater trochanter, parallel to, and 2 cm below, the inguinal ligament. The posterior flap is cut to cover the raw pelvic surface without tension and some of the proximal fibres of the gluteus maximus may be preserved to ensure an adequate blood supply.

The dissection is commenced from the anterior incision and the femoral vessels are ligated and divided first. Then all the anterior and medial groups of muscles are sectioned and the obturator

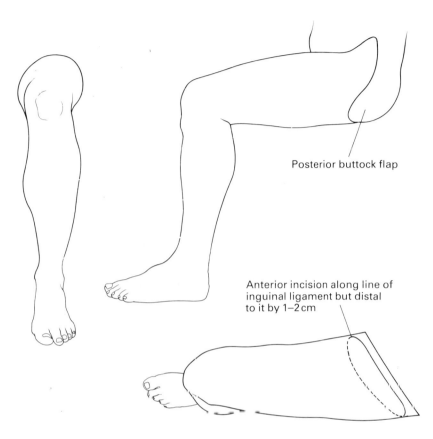

Posterior buttock flap

Anterior incision along line of
inguinal ligament but distal
to it by 1–2 cm

vessels divided between ligatures. The obturator and femoral nerves are divided and the capsule of the hip joint is revealed. Haemostasis in the cut ileopsoas muscle should be obtained while its fibres are being divided, as bleeding may occur after it has retracted into the abdomen.

The anterior capsule of the hip joint is incised and the head of the femur dislocated by externally rotating the leg. This allows the ligamentum teres to be cut and the dislocation is completed so that the posterior aspect of the hip joint can be divided from inside. The sciatic nerve is revealed and divided. The companion artery must be carefully identified and ligated clear of the nerve fibres. Dissection of the posterior flap is completed while the leg is held in a flexed and adducted position by the assistant. The gluteal muscles are divided with ligation of the superior and inferior gluteal vessels. Division of the short muscles around the hip joint frees the specimen. Haemostasis is secured and the flaps approximated with skin stitches only. Suction drainage is provided by the tube drains, one of which must be sited in the acetabulum.

The drains are removed in 48 hours or when drainage ceases. A firm bandage hastens adherence of the flaps and the sutures are removed in 10 to 12 days. The proximity of the anus makes pre-

Fig. 14.3   Disarticulation at the hip. Skin incisions

and postoperative penicillin prophylaxis important and local antibiotic powder or spray before closure of the flaps is desirable.

HINDQUARTER AMPUTATION

This is an amputation of the lower extremity including the hip joint and the related hemipelvis. The absence of the body hemipelvis after hindquarter amputation makes prosthetic replacement an elaborate procedure. Essentially weight is transmitted in the prosthesis via the soft tissues to the sacrum, to the contralateral ischial tuberosity and, to a small degree, to the abdominal contents and thus to the diaphragm and rib cage. This necessitates a large rigid area of body contact in the pelvic region, virtually an exoskeleton, to which the prosthesis can be mounted.

The hindquarter amputation ablates the hemipelvis in the extraperitoneal plane, leaving intact the perineal structures, the sacrum and the extraperitoneal pelvic viscera. The separation of the hemipelvis entails the division of the pubic symphysis and section of the abdominal wall muscles — the external oblique, internal oblique and transverse abdominis — with detachment of the origin of the rectus abdominis. Posteriorly the ileopsoas muscles and quadratus lumborum must be divided while the most medial fibres of gluteus maximus are sectioned subcutaneously together with the piriformis as it crosses the greater sciatic notch.

The perineal structures must be separated from the hemipelvis and this entails division of the sacroiliac ligament, coccygeus and the levator ani muscle diaphragm which is detached from its origin along the obturator internus muscle fascia. Below this the superficial and deep transversus perinei must be detached from the ischial tuberosity, and the compressor urethrae and ishiocavernosus muscles must be separated from the ischial ramus.

At the pelvic brim the common iliac artery and veins are divided together with the trunks amd branches of the sciatic plexus. The branches of the internal iliac artery to the bladder and prostate or the bladder, uterus and vagina are divided. The venous plexus in relation to the prostate and inferior vesical arteries may be responsible for some troublesome bleeding.

Technique

The hindquarter amputation was at one time the most formidable surgical operation in common practice. The technique was described by Hogarth Pringle (1916) and modified by Gordon Taylor and Monroe (1952), who were able to apply the procedure to good result. More recently modern hypotensive anaesthesia and the careful control of circulating blood volume and haemostasis, by careful identification of vessels and the use of diathermy to cut across large masses of muscle, have enabled the operation to be performed even more safely. Our practice follows that described by Westbury (1967).

The patient is placed supine on the operating table. The bladder is catheterized and allowed to drain continuously into a polythene bag away from the operating field. The loin and shoulder on the side for amputation are raised on sandbags and an assistant must be available to hold the leg. A hypotensive technique by the anaesthetist and full muscle relaxation are essential for ease of operation. The incision is made anteriorly and this runs 2 cm above the inguinal ligament from the pubic tubercle to just posterior to the anterior superior iliac spine. Later in the operation the posterior flap is formed and this is preferable to a vertical racquet incision. Once the skin is incised the cutting diathermy point is used to minimize blood loss. The anterior incision is deepened to the peritoneum which enables the peritoneum to be retracted medially, giving access to the iliac vessels in the extraperitoneal plane. Access to these is facilitated by dividing the inferior epigastric vessels and the origin of the rectus abdominis. This also permits clearance of the back of the pubis and enables the subpubic ligament to be divided. The membranous urethra must be safeguarded and venous bleeding controlled with a pack. The symphysis pubis opens once the ligaments are divided and the access to the iliac vessels is considerably improved. The ureter, peritoneum and gonadal vessels are displaced medially by swab dissection.

The common iliac artery is divided between ligatures but the vein must not be ligated until it has been fully cleared. This is not possible until the psoas major has been divided and exposes the sciatic plexus, which must also be divided. Now the iliolumbar veins are revealed which must be individually and carefully ligated to free the common iliac vein, which can then be ligated close to its union with the inferior vena cava. Unless this is done the iliolumbar veins may be avulsed from the common iliac vein with disastrous bleeding. The sacrosciatic notch is then cleared before the posterior skin flap is raised from the gluteal muscles. Some fibres of gluteus maximus may be retained in the posterior flap to facilitate its blood supply unless this compromises the clearance of a tumour.

Once the great sciatic notch is cleared on both sides, a Gigli saw is passed through and the bone cut can be made through either the posterior ileum or the ala of the sacrum. This is preferred to sacro-iliac disarticulation. The remaining structures, obturator internus and piriformis muscles are divided together with the internal iliac vessel branches allowing the specimen to be removed. Any bleeding from the corpus cavernosum or the prostatic venous plexus can be controlled by catgut sutures.

The skin flaps are approximated by skin sutures only and suction tube drainage is used for five to six days. The bladder catheter is removed on the fifth day.

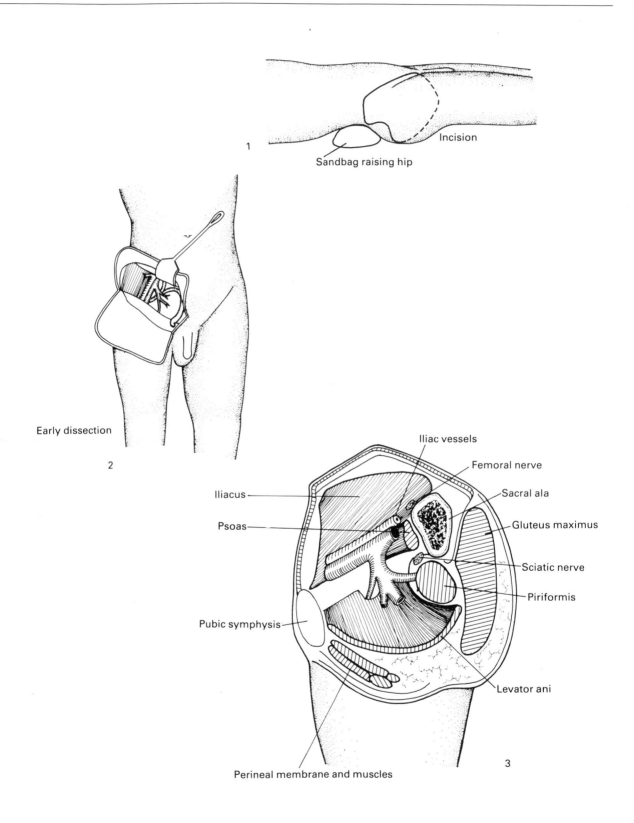

1

Incision

Sandbag raising hip

Early dissection

2

Iliac vessels

Femoral nerve

Sacral ala

Iliacus

Gluteus maximus

Psoas

Sciatic nerve

Piriformis

Pubic symphysis

Levator ani

Perineal membrane and muscles

3

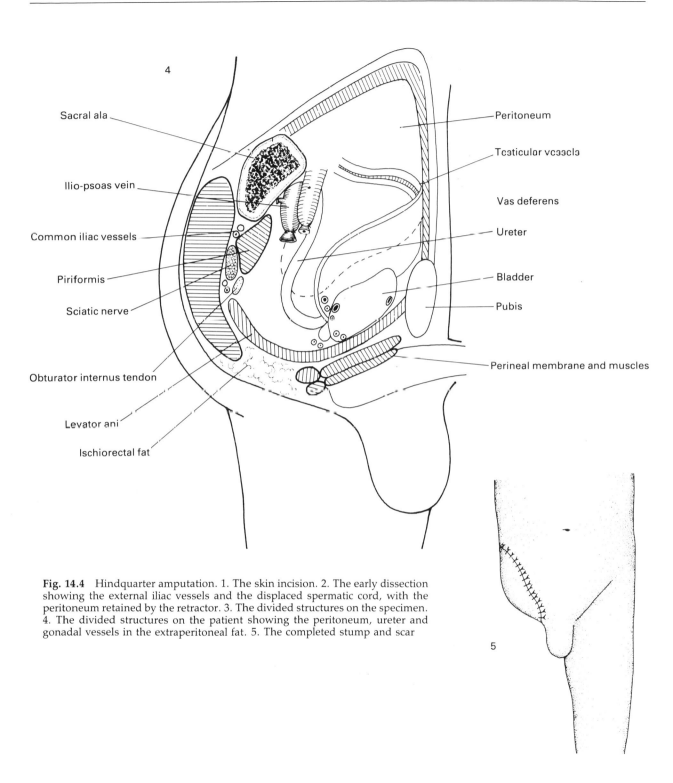

Fig. 14.4   Hindquarter amputation. 1. The skin incision. 2. The early dissection showing the external iliac vessels and the displaced spermatic cord, with the peritoneum retained by the retractor. 3. The divided structures on the specimen. 4. The divided structures on the patient showing the peritoneum, ureter and gonadal vessels in the extraperitoneal fat. 5. The completed stump and scar

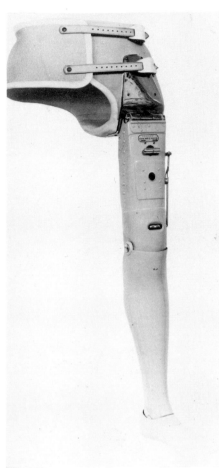

Fig. 14.5   The Canadian tilting table prosthesis for hip disarticulation

PROSTHESES FOR HIP DISARTICULATION

There are two types of prosthesis in use for this level of amputation. One is a legacy from the past and the other was devised by McLaurin of Toronto. The first has a socket which is made to a cast of the pelvis. It is made of any suitable material, such as plastic, blocked leather or metal, and is usually reinforced by metal bands which extend from the midline anteriorly to the midline posteriorly and up to, but not above, the iliac crest. The patient sits in this socket on a sponge rubber or felt pad, taking the weight largely on the ischial tuberosity but also on the buttock muscles and the pelvic wall. This socket is held on to the patient by a waist-belt or by straps running round the opposite side of the pelvis, giving a pull medially to hold the socket onto and under the patient. Suspension over one or both shoulders is usually also required.

In this limb the hip joint is placed directly under the tuber seating. In the sitting position the combined thickness of the socket and the tuber pad of about 2 cm, and the depth of the hip mechanism of 5 cm or more under the ischial tuberosity, prevent the patient from sitting in comfort unless there is a deep half cushion placed under the opposite buttock. It is not surprising that many of these patients prefer to stand. In standing, however, the hip, placed on the vertical line below the centre of gravity, is not in a stable position and therefore has to be locked when walking.

In the second Canadian type of limb, a cast is taken of the whole pelvis. A socket of plastic or blocked leather is made and this embraces the whole pelvis and goes above the iliac crests over which it is closely moulded. In nearly all patients this gives all the suspension needed. The hip joint is placed anteriorly on a line 45° from the vertical from the natural hip joint. There is a sponge rubber or other resilient pad for sitting but this and the wall of the socket are all that are interposed between the ischial tuberosity and the seat. In standing, moreover, the hip joint can be made stable being anterior to the vertical line from the body's centre of gravity.

The older conventional socket is in use principally on patients who are so accustomed to it after years of familiarity that they do not wish to change. It may also have to be used in two types of new amputees. The all-embracing socket of the Canadian type of limb is too restricting for the obese, nor can it be used by them to suspend the limb, so that it may be necessary to give them a conventional socket. This latter socket is also required when the amputation is not a hip disarticulation but a femoral amputation that is too short to make use of a mid-thigh prosthesis. The femoral remnant then flexes and prevents the placing of the hip joint in its anterior position and may require an opening in the socket wall. To place the artificial hip joint in front of this is to make it mechanically too stable and cosmetically unacceptable.

In standing on these sockets there is a significant shift of the centre of gravity towards the opposite leg due to the considerable loss of body weight by amputation. The type of hip joint and its position affects the type of reactions occurring on the stump during walking. In the conventional type of limb, in which the hip joint is locked in full extension, movement is imparted to the prosthesis by movement of the lumbar spine. The rectus abdominis and the anterior lumbar muscles contract strongly to initiate the swing phase by moving the thigh piece, and at the end of the swing phase the erector spinae contracts to decelerate the limb. During the stance phase the erector spinae continues to contract and the lumbar spine becomes lordotic to allow the body to pass over the foot. This produces excessive movement of the lumbar spine which may be acceptable in the young but tends to produce backache in many, thereby limiting their walking distance. In practice therefore many patients tend to wear the socket too loose so that movement can take place between the body and the socket. While this will relieve the lumbar spine of some of its excessive movements it lessens control of the prosthesis, and therefore increases the effort in use. There is also friction which gives rise to problems with the skin.

In this socket therefore there are in the swing phase toe-off pressures acting antero-inferiorly and posterosuperiorly which are reversed at heel contact. Indeed, it is the pressure on the abdominal wall which indicates to the patient the timing of heel contact. During the stance phase the body weight is towards the natural limb and there is therefore a rotating force about the medial edge of the socket. This is counteracted to some extent by body sway but also by the counterpressure of the waist-belt or straps round the contralateral pelvis. Indeed, stability is more easily attained at this level with the short above-knee stump.

With the Canadian type limb the fact that there is hip movement alters the forces involved. During the stance phase the rotating forces due to body weight, body sway, etc. act about the medial border of the socket and are the same except that the all-embracing socket gives firmer, more intimate contact and there is greater stability in the system. It is the anteroposterior forces which are to some extent altered. At heel contact there is pressure on the abdominal wall at the top and on the buttock at the bottom of the socket as the thigh and shin (shank) are decelerated. Because the hip is free to extend it is necessary to keep the hip flexing against its limits to prevent the knee flexing; at this stage the body's weight is acting behind the knee joint while the reaction on the heel is acting in front of the knee joint. As the body passes forward to the mid-stance stage the knee joint becomes inherently stable and the hip extends until it is stopped at full extension. There is then in most versions of this limb a rubber stop, which compresses as the body weight passes over it.

At toe-off the energy absorbed by this compression is first used to initiate the flexion of the knee while the toe is still on the ground and then to impel the thigh and shin (shank) forward in the swing phase. The pressures at the top anteriorly and bottom posteriorly diminish during this process but do not in fact reverse.

During the swing phase the prosthesis swings forward with this rebound assisted to some extent by the effect of gravity on this pendulum. Provided the patient is content to walk at the measured pace of the period of the prosthesis as a pendulum, little other physical effort is required and there is little tendency for there to be movement between the socket and the stump. To attempt to speed up the pace is to expend a lot of energy with little return. To walk faster the hip limits should be adjusted to allow a longer step so that the stride is lengthened with the same periodicity.

A range of free movement at the hip makes the control of knee-shoot at heel contact more difficult for users of this device than for those with the conventional locked hip joint. For some elderly patients a locking knee, such as might have been in the older type of limb, has been necessary. The introduction of stabilizing knees has eliminated this minor disadvantage for most users. The mechanisms at knee and ankle are similar to those at a lower level.

Fig. 14.6 A radiograph showing the body structures remaining after a hindquarter amputation

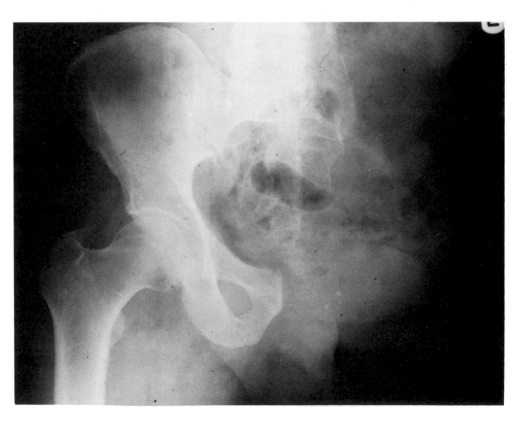

PROSTHESIS FOR HEMIPELVECTOMY

There is no basic difference between the prostheses for use with hindquarter or hemipelvectomy amputations and those used for amputation by disarticulation of the hip. The difference is in the physical qualities of the stump. In disarticulation the whole pelvis with the buttock muscles is firm so that the body's weight can be transmitted almost as if sitting and from which, in modern prostheses, the limb can be suspended. In hemipelvectomy the body's weight must be transmitted to the socket primarily through the abdominal wall, which is enclosing the abdominal contents. These contents are largely a mixture of gas and fluid, with some soft organs such as liver and spleen. The load must therefore be distributed widely and at low pressures to these contents, and the enclosing body wall prevented from distorting. The body contributes the posterior abdominal wall, the opposite side of the pelvis, and the diaphragm which acts as a bulkhead to support the abdominal contents. The socket has to complete the support of the abdominal wall, otherwise the soft tissue will bulge out when a load is applied. It is obvious that diaphragmatic weakness of herniation may be a complication of this amputation. Weakness of the rest of the abdominal wall is also a disadvantage. Also the abdominal contents are not a constant volume, and the amount of gas, which is compressible, is variable.

Therefore the socket for this amputation must complete the encirclement of the abdominal contents and distribute the weight widely over the surface of the abdominal wall. Attempts are sometimes made to gain additional support either from the lower thorax or the contralateral ischial tuberosity. The standard sockets used in the United Kingdom all have a seating crossing the midline to the contralateral ischial tuberosity. Some patients substantiate the claim that when standing still they receive an element of support from this seating.

The transverse seating is not commonly used outside the United Kingdom. Most centres now favour an oblique bearing. The cast for the socket is made with the abdominal contents compressed obliquely so that the lateral wall of the socket is approximately at 45° from the vertical. Whatever the precise theory governing the socket casting it is difficult to prevent some compression of the abdominal contents, some upward displacement of the diaphragm and some extrusion around the edge of the socket. There is also some difficulty in preventing the limb falling away in the swing phase so that it is common to fit this limb somewhat short. The net result is that there is usually a pronounced limp in walking. Nevertheless, many patients lead active lives involving some manual work and there are some young mothers caring for families and managing their own homes without help.

The mechanisms of this prosthesis are identical with those for the hip disarticulation described earlier.

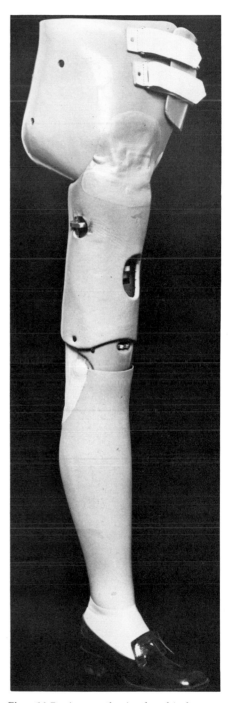

Fig. 14.7 A prosthesis for hindquarter amputation. Note the extended socket floor, reinforced with a metal plate to obtain support from the opposite ischial tuberosity

REHABILITATION

Although immediate prostheses have been supplied to this amputation very successfully this technique is not suitable for general use, and the patient will be encouraged to walk with crutches at the earliest time after operation. When the wound is soundly healed and the contact area is stable, a definitive prosthesis can be constructed.

15

Postoperative Physical and Pathological Changes

Amputation does not guard the stump against the same intercurrent diseases that afflict the normal limb. This chapter is not concerned with such conditions, although they may affect the prosthetic management, nor is it concerned with the inevitable pathology consequent to amputation which has been discussed elsewhere. It is concerned with long-term avoidable pathology of the amputation stump arising from medical or prosthetic practice.

It recognizes that the conditions necessitating amputation, such as trauma, spina bifida etc., may dictate a surgical procedure resulting unavoidably in a stump which is not ideal.

The pathology may be common to many levels of amputation, or specific to one level. Medical causes may arise from uncorrected pre-existing conditions not necessarily associated with the cause of amputation, or from the amputation procedure. Prosthetic causes necessarily arise after amputation. It may be noted that most prosthetic causes will resolve themselves by removal of the prosthesis, although this will not solve the patient's motor and psychological problems, whereas many medical problems continue even when no prosthesis is used.

Medical problems arising from pre-existing pathology are discussed first, followed by generalized problems, both medical and prosthetic, and, finally, medical and prosthetic pathology specific to given levels of amputations.

Short-term pathology arising in the early post-amputation period is not considered, for it either resolves itself, or leads to re-amputation, or develops into the long-term pathology we are considering.

PRE-AMPUTATION PATHOLOGY

Skin

The skin is the body's interface component which has to withstand the forces generated by the use of a prosthesis. Surgery may preserve a useful limb or lead to a more distal amputation but the choice of incision can materially affect the comfort and use of a prosthesis, and the surgeon who is aware that the efforts may not succeed will take into account the possible prosthetic needs, providing they do not jeopardize the procedure that is aimed at preservation.

In vascular surgery, incisions must often be made at a level where the brim of a socket will impinge if amputation becomes necessary, whether at the groin, knee etc. The scar then becomes subjected to the axial pistoning action of the stump and also to rotation of the skeletal elements of the stump within the skin. Vascular surgeons are now much more aware of this and plan their incisions accordingly, but there are still some who are oblivious to the problems they may cause to the patient if amputation becomes necessary.

Scars adherent to the deeper structures, such as may occur following open reduction of fractures, may be acceptable unless amputation, perhaps at a much later date and due to other pathology, requires that limb segment for use with a prosthesis. Some time and trouble taken at the time of amputation in freeing such scarring, so that the skin's mobility over the deeper structures is restored, will add considerably to the patient's comfort.

Plastic surgery will often preserve a useful limb and skin grafts which are not adherent to the skeleton or submitted to high loading are surprisingly successful in retaining a useful distal amputation. It may seem convenient at the time to use the ipsilateral limb as a donor area but should this area need to be part of a higher level of amputation it may give rise to discomfort.

Anaesthetic skin is always a hazard and does not withstand high loading. Unfortunately it cannot always be removed, as in the saddle area present in spina bifida, but unless there is such a specific reason for retaining it, amputation should remove anaesthetic segments.

Fortunately poliomyelitis is now a rare disease in cold and temperate climates so that the severe distressing ulcerating perniosis or chilblains associated with some victims of this disease is no longer common; however, the disease is still endemic in many of the developing third world countries.

Should the surgeon be faced with this problem, he must be wary. Amputation of a flail limb to improve function may be the treatment of choice but if perniosis is the major factor present amputation can be disastrous, for although the skin at a higher level may seem satisfactory at the time, it will develop chilblains after amputation and the patient, who may start with a below-knee amputation, can end up with a disarticulated hip covered with ulcerating, cold skin.

Joints

The pre-amputation state of joints is also important when considering levels of amputation. A flail or unstable joint above an otherwise useful stump is usually acceptable, for a joint can be used in stabilizing prosthetic mechanisms.

When there is active but limited movement in a joint, consideration must be given as to whether the range of movement can be improved and what relation it has to the workload. For example, provided the stump is kept short, amputation below the knee with a flexion deformity of 45° with active movement to

90° at the knee may be acceptable, for the socket can be set in this amount of flexion; whereas if there is a 45° flexion deformity at the hip neither a below-knee nor a knee disarticulation is satisfactory because the knee must be brought vertically below the hip joint when standing, and to achieve this imposes a gross lordosis.

In the upper limb almost any active movement at the wrist, elbow, or shoulder can be used, although a shorter rather than longer stump may be preferred if certain mechanisms which amplify the movement are to be used.

Arthrodesed and ankylosed joints are usually better removed. If retained, the joint cannot be replaced with a prosthetic joint. A disarticulation may then be better. Exception to this is the shoulder if arthrodesed in some abduction and flexion, for this then gives a stable basis from which to operate the prosthesis.

POST-AMPUTATION PATHOLOGY

General (medical)

Skin

There are conventional accepted skin incisions which are based on experience. Unconventional incisions may be imposed by the pathology causing the amputation. New incisions are sometimes introduced and become the new convention when based on anatomical and other studies. Sometimes surgeons devise new incisions with no clear purpose in mind. The latter may sometimes pose a minor embarrassment but in general it can be said that any well-healed skin incision which is freely mobile over the underlying tissues is acceptable.

Skin incisions, however designed, which are adherent to underlying deep tissues, particularly to the skeleton, are a continuing problem, breaking down due to the tension on them in use. Scars at high loading points should be avoided.

Another common fault in fashioning the skin and superficial fascia flaps is to leave redundant tissue. Excessively long flaps below the bone and muscle of the stump prevent the intimate relationship of the socket necessary for stability. These redundant tissues also tend to become oedematous and of poor vascularity. Skin flaps should also be sutured so that 'dog ears' at the ends are not fashioned. They may reduce or disappear in time, but when present they can delay rehabilitation, or in the long-term lead to difficulty in stabilizing the prosthesis on the stump.

Muscles

Modern practice is to reattach muscles as distally as possible and to retain the natural fibre length and alignment. In doing this the agonists and antagonists are usually sutured to each other as well as to the distal end of the bone. Sometimes the attachment to the skeleton is deficient and the opposing groups of muscles move

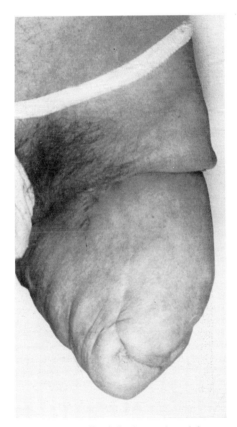

Fig. 15.1 A roll of flesh produced by an ill-fitting above-knee socket

over the bone end. This leads not only to loss of effective power but also to the development of painful bursae, and whether the amputation is by disarticulation or through the shaft of the bone it will normally require operative reattachment.

The muscle flaps in amputations through long bones may also cause prosthetic problems if the whole muscle bulk is sutured over the cut end of bone, for this gives rise to a large bulky mass of muscle and a bulbous stump. Unfortunately such bulbous stumps cannot be used for suspension and there is difficulty in introducing the stump into the socket. Muscles need to be 'tailored' so that the stump, while remaining cylindrical rather than conical, nonetheless has a lesser distal than proximal circumference.

Amputations by the 'guillotine' technique, which may be necessary in infection, as those commonly used after the First World War in which the musculature is allowed to retract, are still practised. Many of these amputations are trouble-free but they frequently produce a stump which can have painful, spasmodic, jactitating muscular contractions. With modern myoplastic amputations they are rarely seen. Such painful spasms can also occur in the non-amputee if there is complete rupture of a muscle belly without repair. The mechanism appears to be the complete retraction of the innervated muscle. Whether revision is desirable depends on the frequency and intensity of the pain. It has been little practised in the United Kingdom but careful removal of the scar tissue and restoration of muscle fibre length with distal attachment was done with considerable success in Germany on some Second World War amputees.

Nerves

The divided nerve heals with a nerve bulb or neuroma despite the various techniques which have been tried, such as crushing, with or without ligation, cauterizing, encapsulating in plastic, muscle, or bone, injection with phenol etc., none of which is successful. The neuroma may be large, exceeding the size of a golf ball, and will be pressed on by the prosthesis, provoking pain. If this occurs exploration of the nerve with higher section and removal of the neuroma becomes necessary. This problem is less frequent than it used to be in these amputations through the use of myoplastic techniques in which the nerve is divided with the least possible trauma and is allowed to retract into the muscle mass. Involvement of the nerve bulb by scar tissue to other structures will produce pain either in the stump or in the phantom bone.

STUMP PATHOLOGY

General (prosthetic)

The skin, as the body's interface, is subjected by the prosthetic interface to forces generated by the prosthesis. The well-fashioned stump should be able to withstand these forces from a well-fitting prosthesis in normal use.

Friction, high pressure, and constriction are all causes of pathological changes in the skin and can usually be overcome by prosthetic changes. Cysts develop in the skin just above the brims of sockets when the skin laps over the edge and is subjected to friction from rotation of the stump within the socket. This is most likely to occur when there is an abrupt change from the socket pressures, and the condition can usually be overcome by bevelling or rounding the socket edge so that there is a more gradual transition from the higher socket pressure to no pressure at all. These cysts, originally considered to be sebaceous cysts but now regarded by many to be inclusion dermoid cysts due to repeated impact, are particularly difficult when they occur in the groin. They were common when the plug-fit type of socket for thigh amputation was used. When they occur in modern sockets it will nearly always be due to there being too little room in the adductor region, for example if the amputee has put on weight, as well as to faulty fitting by the prosthetist. If not overcome by prosthetic refit at an early stage, they may become infected and require surgical removal. Similar infected cysts may sometimes develop in the axilla due to the harness for the operating cord or suspension. It may be overcome by changing the materials used, but if persistent may require an alternative method of suspension and a different method of pulling on the operating cord.

High loading at the upper and lower extremes of the stump may be due to the amputee's heavy use of the prosthesis, causing

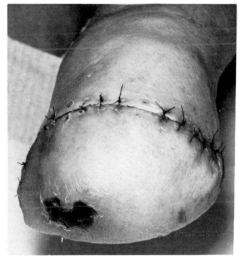

Fig. 15.2 Pressure necrosis in a below-knee stump

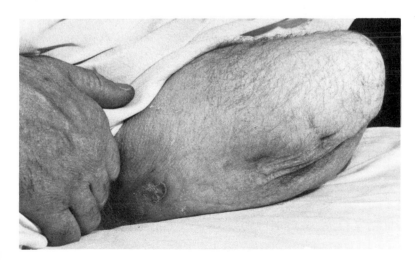

Fig. 15.3 Septic epidermoid cysts in an above-knee stump

transverse forces beyond the tolerance of the skin. In the upper limb the major loading in use of the prosthesis will commonly be such forces, and if they are intermittent they will be tolerated. The sustained load, as when holding a welder's shield on the forearm, is the kind of force which can give rise to painful skin conditions. In the lower limb the driving position with the foot on the accelerator may produce a similar problem. A socket which fits intimately and distributes the load proximally may be all that is required. If this does not overcome the problem the addition of an upper-arm corset with side steels and a locking elbow-joint may overcome the upper-limb problem, and an elastic pick-up to a waist-belt may overcome the driving problem.

Similar pressure areas also arise from prosthetic alignment in the lower limb. In the stance phase of gait the foot should be under the centre of body mass. A fairly common fault is for the prosthetist to set the foot too far from the midline. The ground reaction is then directed laterally to the knee joint causing, in the below-knee amputee, pressure on the fibular head and gaping on the medial side of the socket. Occasionally the foot is misplaced medially with similar reversed pathology. Similar malalignment of the foot may cause excessive pressure on the lateral aspect distally of the thigh amputation.

Lastly there are discoloration, skin oedema, and eczema of the distal part of the stump due to the circumferential pressure proximally and the unsupported superficial tissues, as has been described in the chapter on 'Principles of Prosthetic Design'. That it does not occur more often is due to the support afforded by the stump socks and, when the socket is closed, the pneumatic cushion of air in the socket chamber. It is often precipitated by the amputee putting on weight and forcing the stump into a socket which is then too tight. It can be cured by steps being taken to reduce the circumferential pressures, e.g. using thin stump socks or renewing the socket, and by adding a soft-tissue supporting touch-pad of any suitable material, such as lamb's wool, plastic foam, etc. Although this will overcome the basic condition, the discoloration may remain as a permanency.

Because the prosthesis can only affect the body tissues through the skin, deeper tissues are less likely to be affected by the prosthesis, except joints and bone.

The loss of symmetry in the upper limb tends, in the long term, to produce a scoliosis, a tendency which is further encouraged by the wearing of a prosthetic harness and using an operating cord. The long-term use of a single shoulder suspension for lower-limb prostheses also encourages the development of a scoliosis. Modern techniques of suspension have reduced this tendency.

Lower limb amputations

Through ankle

Surgical causes. Amputation at the ankle at the preferred level

may develop pathology even when the bone section is at the joint. It is important that the heel pad should become firmly adherent to the cut end of bone otherwise in use it may become displaced. It is also important that the bone section should be horizontal with the ground which may make it necessary to have some obliquity to the tibial shaft if there is bowing of the tibia. If it is not horizontal the heel pad will usually migrate to one side in active use. Sometimes the Achilles tendon may be attached to the heel pad and this will distract it from its terminal position. These are complications which may occur in the ankle amputation as described by Syme.

Prosthetic causes. The well-fitting prosthesis does not give rise to stump pathology and even the ill-fitting one rarely does. As with any prosthesis there are some inherent problems, which at this level is the provision of ankle movement and the bulky ankle. These problems have largely been overcome in the prosthesis. Unhappily over the years many surgeons have tried to overcome these prosthetic problems surgically. These amputations are not Syme's but modifications which usually result in an amputation which is really an over-long below-knee amputation.

Bauden's tibiotarsal amputation, described in 1842, and Guyon's supramalleolar amputation are earlier variants, but it was Elmslie's modification in 1924 which has been most commonly used in recent years. More recently, Wagner has introduced a two stage modification.

In Elmslie's amputation the tibia and fibula were transected at a level well above the ankle joint, thereby (a) impairing or destroying the anastomosis in the distal growth plate scars, (b) causing the heel flap to be smaller and from the posterior aspect of the heel rather than the heel pad itself, (c) reducing the effective load-bearing area by half, (d) removing the bulbous nature of the stump and therefore its self-suspending properties. Few of these amputations are able to sustain the full end-bearing load. The stumps are often ischaemic and ulcerating and proximal load-bearing becomes essential, as is auxiliary suspension.

The two-stage amputation follows the original technique in the first instance, using the heel pad; in the secondary stage the malleoli are trimmed vertically. This provides better vascularity and the heel flap is better adapted for weight-bearing but there is still a reduction in the area available, leading to an increase in the unit loading on the stump, and the prosthesis is no longer self-suspending.

Below-knee levels

Most stump pathology is due to one of the common factors — malalignment, adherent scars, etc. — discussed earlier. There are a few examples of specific pathology.

Surgical. In the preferred amputation with the long posterior flaps too little attention can be given to the contours of the cut bone end. This is in part due to earlier textbooks emphasizing the need to 'bevel' the cut end of tibia. This is preferable to a transverse section of bone but is not enough. With a transverse section there is a sharp anterior edge to the tibia which is subcutaneous and difficult to protect from the prosthetic socket. To bevel the tibia reduces, but does not eliminate, the sharp anterior edge, and adds two other sharp edges. Rounding the contours of the tibia and fibula at amputation, as advocated, provides a bone end which is acceptable.

Another bone problem occurs in the osteomyoplastic amputation, described by Jackson Burrows, Loon, Dederich and others in which there is a bony bridge fashioned between the tibia and fibula. Even after it has apparently become successful it may in time undergo various pathological changes such as osteoporosis, stress fracture, aseptic necrosis, etc. Conservative treatment may be successful but takes a long time. As these stumps are usually longer, a quicker solution may be to revise the amputation to the shorter posterior flap.

Long below-knee amputation stumps, such as may occur with guillotine amputations in trauma, are at a level which has poor skin vascularity and little or no muscular tissue to insulate the bone from the prosthesis. These long stumps are usually the result of the amputee refusing the intended revision once the sepsis has been overcome.

Prosthetic. The PTB socket, which is the type of socket commonly used at this level of amputation, can give rise to some problems. The original concept of taking the major load on the patellar tendon when done as it was conceived will not usually give rise to problems, although modern practice is not to make such a deep bar as was originally described. The patellar bar can give rise to excessive pressure if it is too deep and the other high-loading areas are not being effectively used. But the major problem is too wide a bar which impinges on the edge of the tibial plateau.

The other prosthetic problem specific to this area is caused by the medial hamstrings. As insertion of the medial hamstrings into the tibia is variable, the posterior brim of the socket needs to be lowered to allow for this tendon in flexion of the knee.

Amputation at the knee

Surgical. Surgical amputation at the knee by disarticulation using lateral flaps has no inherent problem liable to give rise to stump pathology. There may be, as at other levels, inadequate skin flaps or failure to attach the musculature distally. For some time the skin flaps were fashioned as a long anterior flap extending well below the tibial tubercle, which led, in too many cases, to an area of skin necrosis. This incision is no longer advocated.

Prosthetic. There are no inherent difficulties giving rise to stump pathology from the prosthesis.

Other amputations near to the knee joint

1. Short below-knee.

Surgical. Unless there is a tibial remnant long enough to give some leverage to a below-knee type of prosthesis, the knee must be flexed so that the load is taken as in kneeling. Some surgeons do such amputations in preference to a knee disarticulation. Provided the surgery is well done there is no inherent surgical pathology to this amputation apart from the fact that it imposes the use of a knee-disarticulation type of prosthesis with some additional prosthetic disadvantages.

Prosthetic. The flexed knee stump projecting backwards imposes the use of a socket into which the thigh and knee stump must be introduced through a front opening, and prevents the use of the modern push-in socket.

This amputation also has two pathological conditions not found in the knee disarticulation. The load is transmitted through the flexed knee, as in kneeling, and a pre-patellar bursitis may develop, which can become chronic. The second problem arises from reflex movement of the below knee stump which may cause friction between the stump and socket; this may be difficult to overcome in the prosthesis.

2. Modification above the knee joint.

The modifications to the knee-disarticulation amputation are too numerous to describe in detail. They mostly attempt to improve the cosmetic appearance of the prosthesis and can be divided into three major categories:

(a) those retaining the patella in its natural position
(b) those transposing the patella to the end of the femur
(c) those which remove the patella

(a) Those retaining the patella in position. Some surgeons, while doing the standard procedure, have tried to improve the cosmesis by vertical section of both femoral condyles. This results in a loss of cross-section and increases the unit load at the end of the stump.

These amputations retain an element of end-bearing but usually need some proximal load-bearing. They also destroy the self-suspension by the socket. There is also impairment of the collateral circulation through the geniculate arteries.

Another variant has been the transcondylar amputation. Although these heal readily and initially can take full end-bearing, they eventually are unable to take the full load and develop vascular problems.

(b) Those transposing the patella to the femoral end. There are many variants of these amputations, usually given the title 'Gritti–Stokes'. These are the bane of the prosthetist. The concept was to transpose the patella to the cut end of the femur at a level where the cross-section of the femur matched the patella. Some surgeons have advocated a lower section through the condyles but are still attaching the patella below the condyles. These

amputations heal readily but give rise to many problems. The patella can be avulsed from its attachment by the quadriceps, it can become osteoporotic, and it can undergo aseptic necrosis. The patella is a sesamoid bone and its architecture is not designed for impact, nor is the skin, which in these amputations is at the end of the stump. There is frequently an imbalance between hip flexors and extensors leading to a hip flexion deformity. There is also frequently impaired circulation leading to severe vascular pain. Many of these amputees cannot wear a prosthesis because of these complications, and those that do have to wear one take much or even all of the load proximally, as in a thigh amputation.

(c) Amputation with removal of patella. If the condyles are left intact they are usually end-bearing but have no advantages over knee disarticulation, and the loss of the patella makes control of rotation more difficult. If there is other surgery, it adds many of the difficulties of the Gritti–Stokes' amputation.

Prosthetic. There is no prosthetic pathology which is not generated by the surgery.

Above-knee amputation

Surgical. There is no common pathology peculiar to this level of amputation although it suffers more than most levels from the surgical problems common to all levels, such as being over-long, too short, leaving infolded scars, etc.

Prosthetic. This level of amputation gives rise to prosthetic pathology, but again it is largely the same as that caused by prostheses at other levels, although it is encountered more frequently at this level.

Amputation at the hip

Surgical. When amputation at the hip is done as described, pathological sequelae are rare. Unfortunately the conditions giving rise to such amputations, such as trauma, neoplasm, or vascular gangrene, may impose modifications to the amputation technique.

The major surgical cause of difficulty is in fact the over-short thigh amputation in which the femoral stump does not project below the pubic ramus sufficiently to fit a prosthesis. The femoral stump adopts a flexed abducted position which prevents the modern hip mechanisms being used and makes it necessary to modify the socket to accommodate this remnant. It can then be difficult to prevent the socket moving on the stump, thus giving rise to soreness.

Prosthetic. There are no prosthetic causes of pathology peculiar to this level of amputation. Poor fit and alignment, as at other levels, give rise to discomfort and friction.

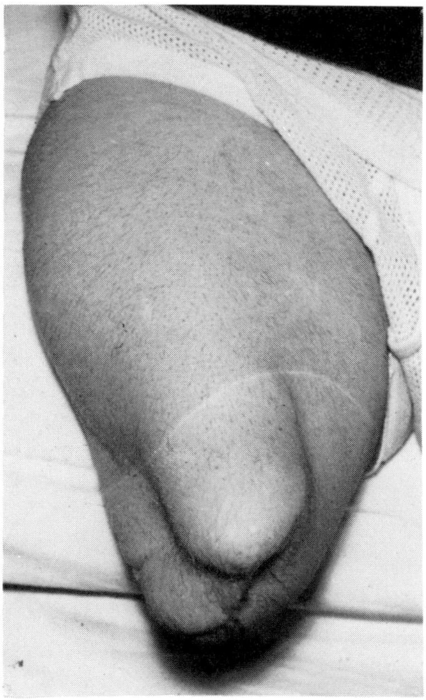

Fig. 15.4 An unsupported femoral stump protruding through the skin forming terminal ulceration

Amputation through the pelvis

The prosthesis used for this amputation is similar to that used for hip disarticulation and its problems are similar.

There is one problem which is inevitable. In this amputation the load has to be taken largely by as wide a distribution as possible on the abdominal contents, a gas and fluid mixture, which is compressed in the stance phase. It is therefore inevitable that these patients have a considerable limp, of which they will sometimes complain. Injudicious sympathetic remarks by those not familiar with the cause of the problem may then fan the amputees' dissatisfaction beyond alleviation.

UPPER LIMBS

Avoidable pathology peculiar to specific levels of amputation is not a feature of upper-limb amputations. Such problems as arise are those discussed in the General section, such as injudicious incisions in areas subject to high load, retention of anaesthetic skin, etc., on the surgical side, and poor fit of the socket or friction from harness by the prosthesis.

16

Management of Congenital Deformities

THE UPPER LIMB

Below-elbow

Excluding malformations of fingers and hands the commonest limb deficiency is absence of the distal two-thirds of the forearm and hand, the left limb being affected twice as often as the right. The stump end is rounded and usually bears minute digital rudiments (Fig. 16.1). These indicate that the condition is a failure of development and *not* a congenital amputation (a condition of extreme rarity).

The vast majority of limb deficiencies are not hereditary and are never likely to recur in siblings and children of those affected.

Prostheses

A one-piece forearm and foam hand with a lifelike plastic glove covering should be supplied between the sixth and eighth month. It is recommended that both parents attend an Artificial Limb and Appliance Centre within a week or two of the child's birth so that a future programme can be outlined. At the same

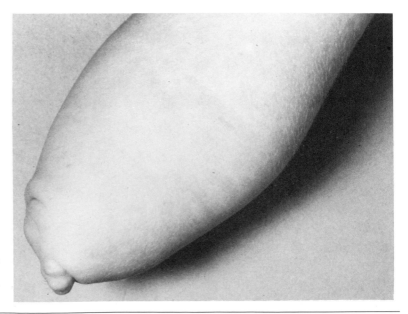

Fig. 16.1 Congenital below-elbow deficiency. Note the rudimentary crest of digital buds. From G.T. McCarthy (1984), with kind permission of the publishers, Faber and Faber

time reassurance may be given about additions to the family, schooling and upbringing, etc. At about 18 months of age the child should be prescribed a functional limb and in due course a myoelectric prosthesis may be offered. As the latter is quite heavy it is rare to fit one to a child under 3.5 years of age.

Frequent periods of instruction in the use of a prosthesis are given to children during the growing years.

Absence of the hand (acheiria)

This is the second commonest deficiency. Apart from being thinner the forearm appears to be relatively normal and possesses full elbow movement and rotation. A strong wrist, often with a proximal palmar rudiment, exists although carpal bones are deficient and may not be evident on X-ray for many years. As the child grows the forearm is noted to be approximately 1.5 cm shorter than its fellow. The stump end has sensation comparable with that of a normal finger tip.

Treatment

Because of the exquisite tactile sensibility a prosthesis should *not* be prescribed.

Illogical as it may seem parents must be assured that their child will have only a negligible handicap and that the normal free use of the limb is the best solution. There are many people with absence of both hands who lead perfectly normal lives; they can dress, fasten buttons, eat, write, etc., completely unaided.

One slight problem is that of using two eating utensils. This is overcome, on the left side, by supplying a simple wrist-band which is made of light leather, about 4 cm wide, and is secured by two narrow straps and buckles. A fork may then be slid between the band and the volar aspect of the wrist (Fig. 16.2). When the

Fig. 16.2 Dinner-fork held by broad leather wrist band. From G.T. McCarthy (1984), with kind permission of the publishers, Faber and Faber

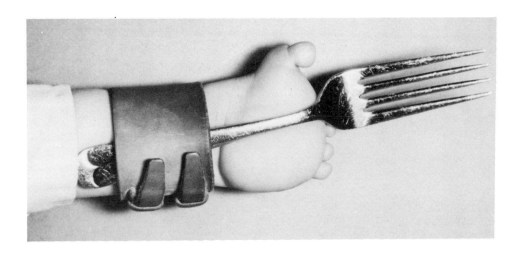

right hand is missing and a knife is required to be held, the band is supplied with a slot and a pocket in which the handle lodges. For very young children, learning how to use a knife, it is advisable to rotate the blade 90° on the handle. Once the skill in using the implement has been acquired an ordinary knife can be used confidently.

During the early teens the child may request a cosmetic hand for social reasons and this can be supplied. It is usually discarded when confidence has been established and the youngster realizes that members of the opposite sex are not adversely affected by the deficiency.

Some babies are born with absence of the hand and a forearm three-quarters the normal length. In such instances the stump is usually tapered and the wrist rudiment very poorly formed. Although it is advisable to fit a prosthesis (as mentioned above for the short below-elbow deficiency), the parents should be warned that it may be rejected. Only about 40% of children with these rather long tapered stumps accept an artificial limb.

The transfer of one or more toes to a digitless hand has been advocated by some plastic surgeons but it is a practice abhorred by clinicians specializing in limb deficiencies. It ruins natural function, constitutes a dual handicap (since a foot is mutilated) and psychological problems ensue because of the appearance of the hand. People with malformed or mutilated fingers are far more self-conscious than those with a neat rounded stump. Appearance far outweighs functional handicap which, in the congenital hand deficiencies, is minimal.

Absence at or above-elbow

As isolated deficiencies these two levels of hemimelia are quite rare. They are usually accompanied by bilateral lower-limb defects and experience has shown that children very rarely accept more than two prostheses. If, therefore, both lower limbs are fitted with prostheses none should be supplied to the upper! If *only* an arm is affected then a one-piece cosmetic limb, with a slightly flexed elbow, should be supplied at about one year of age. An activated prosthesis with a friction elbow joint may be given at about 20–24 months.

Complete absence of the arm (amelia)

This is a very rare phenomenon as a single entity. Bilateral amelia is slightly less rare. Sometimes a single flail digit is present at the right shoulder (Fig. 16.3). This should *not* be removed nor should stabilization be attempted.

Treatment

Whether unilateral or bilateral, prostheses should not be supplied. However sophisticated they are (or may become) they

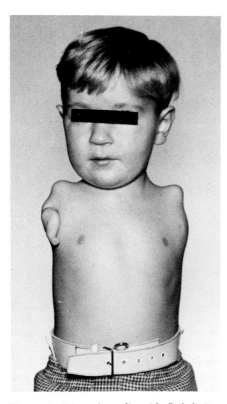

Fig. 16.3 Bilateral amelia with flail digit at the right shoulder

prevent the child from engaging in the normal rough and tumble of school and pre-school life. It is unrealistic to expect either a parent or teacher to remove the limb(s) for play and then don them and redress the child. Frustration is inevitable.

Those with bilateral amelia and normal lower limbs become so dextrous with their prehensile feet that ultimately they become completely independent. Many such adults live normal lives, drive cars, engage in a variety of sports, marry and have normal children.

Phocomelia

This is the name given to a very short 'flipper-like' limb in which the hand or foot is at or near the shoulder and hip respectively (Fig. 16.4). In the case of the upper limb there is nearly always one long bone present and this is almost invariably the ulna. Since the humerus is missing the shoulder joint is non-existent and only minimal active abduction is possible.

Treatment

Surgery is contraindicated. Attempts to stabilize the shoulder have, in the past, proved fruitless. Nevertheless, people with bilateral phocomelia do manage to lead near-normal lives. Some, like the bilateral amelics, use their feet for prehension. Prostheses should *not* be attempted for the bilaterally affected but may be considered for a unilateral defect. The socket should be made of leather with an appropriate aperture for the little hand and the prosthesis is otherwise similar to that made for an above-elbow amputee.

Cleft hand (lobster-claw hand)

This condition is often bilateral and associated with a similar deformity of the feet. It is one of the very few limb anomalies which is known to be hereditary (Fig. 16.5).

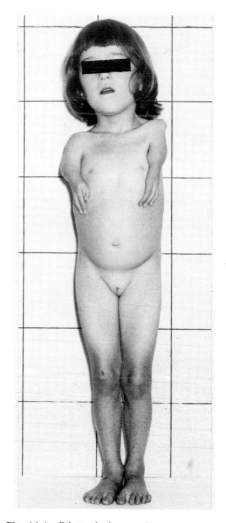

Fig. 16.4 Bilateral phocomelia

Treatment

The hands have excellent function because of their extremely wide spread. Psychological problems may lead to a request for surgery, in which case closure of the cleft should be considered. As with other types of surgery on children's hands the older the subject the better the result. However, the longer the delay the more difficult it is for the person to adapt to the altered hand shape. For this reason it is advisable to plan the closure during the first decade.

Ring constrictions

The cause of these limb conditions is obscure. They have been attributed to amniotic bands but this is viewed with some scepticism. There has also been the suggestion that an abortifacient is responsible but evidence is, for obvious reasons, lacking.

Fig. 16.5 Cleft (lobster-claw) hands combined with gross lower-limb malformations

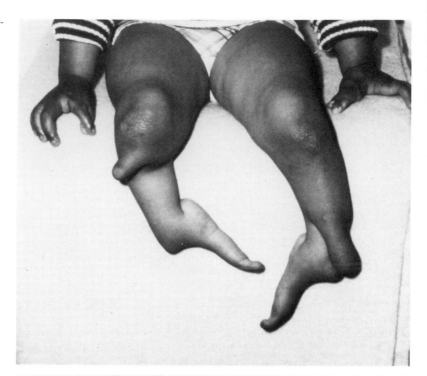

(a)

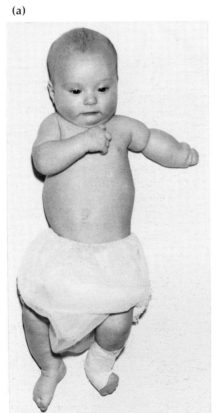

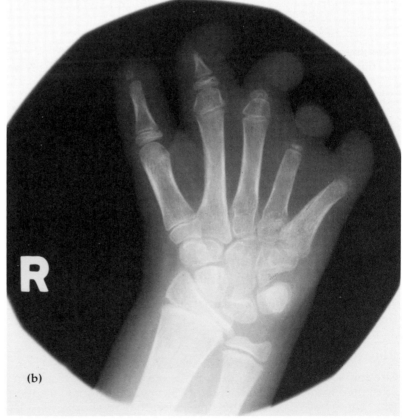

Fig. 16.6 Ring constrictions of (a) left arm and wrist — note lower limb anomaly, (b) fingers — note absence of bone distal to the lesions

It is usual for more than one limb to be affected, often the main segment, also fingers and toes. When the digits are involved there is no bone distal to the constriction bands and some of the tips may possibly be absent. The limb with a constriction band has a gross appearance of a tight cord embedded in oedematous flesh. No actual ligature is present at birth as the constriction is subcutaneous (see Fig. 16.6).

Treatment

When a flail, insensitive distal segment of an arm or leg exists amputation is advisable and should be followed by standard prosthetic fitting.

THE LOWER LIMB

Congenital defects of the lower limb are comparatively rare. On their own they account for 19% of all dysmelias. The percentage of malformations confined to the upper limbs is 63%, and those affecting upper *and* lower limbs is 18%.

Transverse terminal deficiencies, as *single* entities, are extremely rare. They do, however, occur bilaterally and then they are often associated with an upper-limb anomaly. They are not, and should not be referred to as congenital amputations.

Treatment

Standard prostheses, as for an amputation, should be supplied with a simple knee joint, as no mechanisms are included before the teens. Ankle joints are also unnecessary until about 8 or 10 years of age.

The most frequently occurring lower-limb anomaly is a dysplasia resulting in gross limb shortening. This may be confined to: (a) the femur; (b) the tibia; or (c) both.

(a) Short or absent femur

Although there are a variety of femoral dysplasias (almost invariably proximal and occasionally complete aplasia exists), there are two main types which are of practical concern:
1 those with a stable hip
2 those with an absent or unstable hip

In both types the leg often has a reasonably normal tibia and fibula, with a well-formed foot possessing five toes (even when the femur is completely absent).

Treatment

When considerable shortening exists an extension prosthesis is indicated.

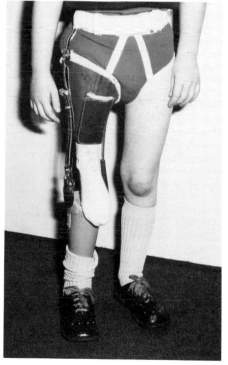

Fig. 16.7 Extension prosthesis fitted for absence of the femur. The foot is unsupported. From G.T. McCarthy (1984), with kind permission of the publishers, Faber and Faber

Stable hip joint

The prosthesis need only extend to the knee, while the foot is set in a comfortable degree of equinus in a blocked leather bootee, set on a platform with metal side struts. These are joined posteriorly by a steel calf band. Depending upon the amount of equinus achieved it may be possible to accommodate the foot and leg within a metal-enclosed prosthesis.

Unstable hip joint.

A prosthesis with ischial tuber bearing is essential and is achieved by having a snugly fitted blocked leather open-ended socket. This is made from a cast of the whole limb. A platform should not be incorporated, otherwise telescoping will occur at the hip as growth proceeds. Instead the foot is allowed to hang free (Fig. 16.7). Metal side struts, riveted to the socket, extend down to an artificial shin and foot, and a rigid pelvic band with a hip joint, as fitted to standard artificial limbs, is usually necessary. An encircling strap placed around the natural foot and side steels affords sufficient anchorage for the child to control the prosthesis when walking and running. Many youngsters so fitted engage in football and various other sporting activities.

Surgery

When there is gross shortening and the foot is either level with, or slightly above, the contralateral knee joint, a disarticulation at the ankle may be contemplated and a reasonably conventional prosthesis fitted.

It should be appreciated, however, that a severe degree of proximal femoral dysplasia is frequently associated with a fixed flexion contracture of the hip and knee. Removal of the foot without correction of the contractures will be fraught with disaster. Soft-tissue surgery of the popliteal area may be inadequate and therefore an arthrodesis of the knee will be required. Careful planning and growth estimation are essential.

Van Nes Procedure.

This is an operation which is sometimes performed when the foot on the affected limb is level with the contralateral knee. A tibial rotation osteotomy of 180° is performed, thus bringing the heel and sole of the foot to the front. A modified below-knee prosthesis, with thigh corset and side steels, is then fitted. The heel gives the appearance of a knee and the foot acts as a below-knee stump. When performed on children derotation occurs and the procedure needs to be repeated (Fig. 16.8). Meanwhile great difficulty is experienced in using the prosthesis. The appearance of the rotated limb is so bizarre that the child is likely to avoid swimming and other activities which entail the removal of the prosthesis. Psychological effects in a number of children have only been solved by subsequent amputation of the foot.

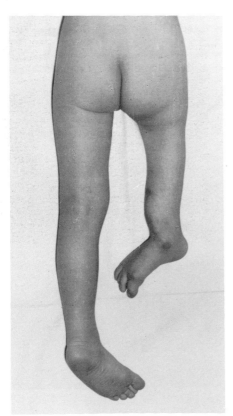

Fig. 16.8 De-rotation which occurred within two years following Van Nes procedure

(b) Short tibia

This is usually associated with an absent fibula (fibular hemimelia). Not only is the tibia short but it is bowed anteriorly and has a longitudinal dimple adherent to the apex of the kyphos (Fig. 16.9). Very occasionally there is radiological evidence of a pseudarthrosis but it is very unwise to attempt a bone graft unless there is demonstrable movement.

When the fibula is absent the lateral one or two rays of the foot are also missing. The majority of infants born with this defect have an everted foot, which if left in situ will inevitably result in poor cosmesis (Fig. 16.10).

Treatment

When the foot is everted removal at the ankle level is an ideal solution. A simple disarticulation, but not the Syme procedure, should be performed, at or before the tenth month and the prosthesis fitted by the first year. If shortening is considerable the stump is fitted as for a below-knee amputation, i.e. a plastic shin and a flexible foot. In the rare event of the foot lying in line with the long axis of the tibia and if the overall shortening is greater than the length of the foot, an extension prosthesis can be fitted (Fig. 16.11). The foot is naturally in some degree of equinus, due to a very tight Achilles tendon, and full equinus should be attempted, probably in stages. A platform prosthesis is supplied initially but later a fully enclosed type is used and this provides excellent cosmesis.

Leg lengthening

When the amount of shortening is not excessive but insufficient to permit the fitting of an extension prosthesis, consideration should be given to a lengthening procedure. It is very important, however, that the foot will be plantigrade and able to take full and painless weight-bearing. It is also essential that both shoes are the same size, since some parents and adult patients have complained about having to wear odd sizes or even surgical footwear.

Many a young person would favour an amputation in order to wear normal shoes in preference to having an unsightly and possibly uncomfortable foot.

Before an irrevocable decision is reached about the treatment of a short lower limb there should be a consultation at an Artificial Limb and Appliance Centre.

Phocomelia

This is another rare anomaly which may be either unilateral or bilateral and many thalidomide victims have the latter.

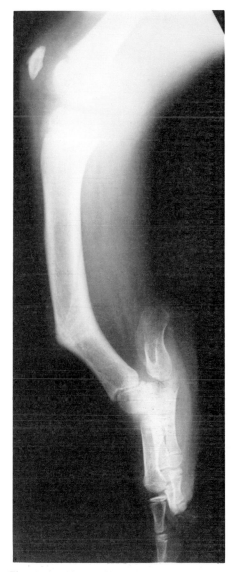

Fig. 16.9 Absent fibula — short tibia with anterior bowing and foot in equinus

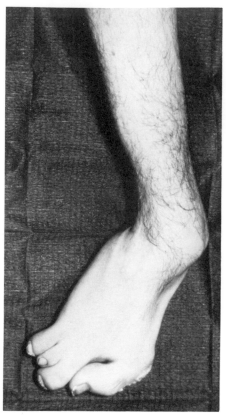

Fig. 16.10 Absent fibula — everted foot with absent lateral ray

Treatment

If unilateral, an extension prosthesis should be fitted, with an open-ended blocked leather socket kept high on the outer side to embrace most of the buttock. The foot should be unsupported, as already described above. The early prosthesis should have a rigid-type pelvic band incorporated, although it may be possible to dispense with this when the child is older. Teenagers object to the excessive width of their hips if they have a pelvic band, saying 'Jeans cannot be worn'!

Unlike an above-knee amputee the thigh and hip area of a phocomelic is much more prominent. There is, of course, no hip joint and the person walks with a marked Trendelenburg gait and exaggerated arm swing.

On *no* account should the diminutive foot be amputated. Flail as the limb may be, the foot is a good anchor for the prosthesis and provides the necessary leverage for walking.

At about six months of age a baby with bilateral phocomelia should be fitted with a device known as a 'sitting socket'. This completely embraces both hips and has apertures through which the feet protrude. The socket is then mounted on a toy dog which, in turn, is secured to a 43 cm square platform under which

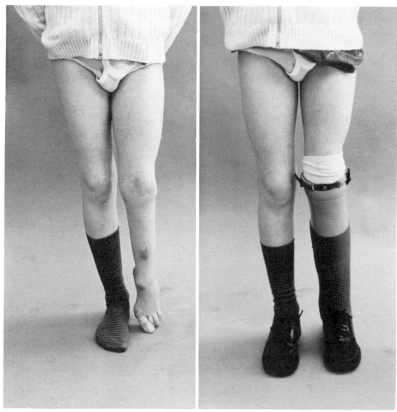

Fig. 16.11 Absent fibula — (a) equinus foot in line with tibia, (b) leg fully enclosed in extension prosthesis

(a)   (b)

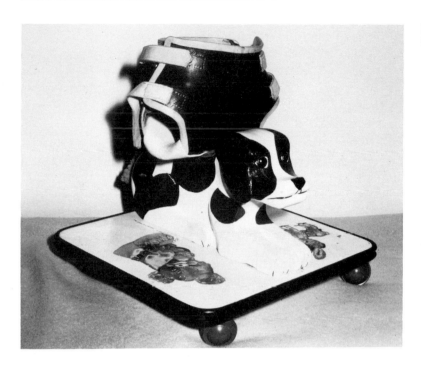

Fig. 16.12   'Sitting socket' with apertures for feet, mounted on wooden dog on casters

four castors are fitted (Fig. 16.12). At approximately one year of age a device known as 'swivel walkers' should be substituted. This is a Canadian invention of the mid-60s which has proved very useful for bilateral phocomelics and amelics. The non-articulated legs are attached to a spring-loaded mechanism fixed under the platform on which the double-sided socket is mounted. The feet make floor contact only on their inner edges as the soles are canted 15° to give a minimal amount of eversion. When the child tilts gently to one side the foot then lies flat on the floor and the other one lifts clear. Rotating the body towards the side of the supporting foot causes the whole device to swivel, thus bringing the other leg forward. Tilting the body to the opposite side results in a repeat performance and allows the child to progress at quite a reasonable rate without any other external aid. The ground must be completely flat and horizontal because no form of slope or step can be negotiated.

In due course, a separate prosthesis for each limb is provided but crutches or sticks may then be required, particularly for the bilateral amelic who progresses by means of a tripod gait at quite a fast speed.

People with phocomelia are supplied with extension prostheses and those with bilateral amelia are given non-jointed hip disarticulation-type limbs. These are comparatively lighter than the articulated limbs.

Hip and knee joints may be added when there is a strong demand by the patient but the extra weight is a factor to be considered.

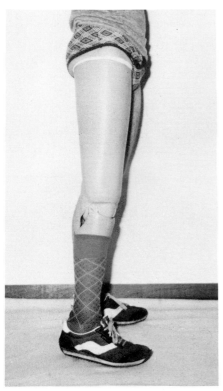

Fig. 16.13 Prosthesis supplied after through-knee amputation for absent tibia

Absence of the tibia (tibial hemimelia)

A child born with absence of the tibia usually has a fairly normal foot which is grossly inverted, due to the lack of ankle mortice and presence of the fibula, the upper end of which retains its fetal position at the outer side of the lateral femoral condyle.

Treatment

Over the years a variety of operations have been performed in an attempt to preserve such limbs but none is as satisfactory as amputation at the knee. This should be performed well before the first birthday so that a prosthesis can be supplied at that time. A child growing up with such an amputation and prosthesis can lead a perfectly ordinary life (Fig. 16.13). Some are known to play football, volley-ball and to run with negligible limp. To delay the amputation until the child is in its teens will result in a poorer performance and deprive it of a near-normal childhood.

The prosthesis for the infant is non-articulated but is complete with a foot, rigid ankle and flexible pelvic band. Although the socket encases the thigh, full end-bearing is taken on the stump end. At about the age of two years, a knee joint is provided without a lock, and the child adapts very quickly to free-knee walking and should then be treated in the same way as his peers.

Parents should not be alarmed if they find the youngster on a climbing-frame or up a tree!

17
Future Developments

The first chapter outlined the development of amputation surgery and external limb prosthetics through the ages to the present day. The main body of the book is concerned with the incidence and causes of amputation in the United Kingdom, the principles of amputation surgery and the management of the postoperative period, and the principles of the use of external prosthetic replacement of limbs, and social integration.

The art and practice of medicine are not static. This last chapter speculates on the likely changes in amputation surgery and prosthetic limb replacement in the next few years, which may be considered under three headings, namely prevention, alternative treatment, and new amputation and prosthetic techniques.

PREVENTION

Our understanding of the causes of congenital deformities, whether genetic or due to noxious substances, is advancing. The identification of drugs responsible for these deformities is expanding and techniques for the diagnosis of deformities in utero has made the incidence of such deformities more preventable, so hopefully their incidence in the population will decrease. However, the worldwide improvement in the delivery of health care may lead for a time to a high survival rate, particularly of the more severely deformed.

Trauma has long been associated with amputation and is still thought by laymen to be the major cause of amputation. This is no longer so in Westernized countries except in wartime. Unhappily, wars and terrorism are still prevalent in many parts of the world and prevention depends on political decisions rather than medical advances. Industrial and traffic accidents are responsible for much of the other traumatic amputations and these could be reduced by governments introducing and enforcing preventive measures.

In Europeanized societies vascular disease is now the commonest cause of amputation, whereas it is still a minor cause in other cultures with a high standard of living, such as the Japanese. As more is known about the causes of vascular disease, diet, smoking, stress, exercise, etc., propaganda may alter habits and reduce the incidence of vascular disease. Unhappily, many cultures hitherto free are now adopting European habits and are reporting a higher incidence of vascular disease. Worldwide, therefore, there may be an increase in vascular disease, particularly where expectation of life has been raised rather than reduced. Diabetes, both in its neurological and its vascular manifestation, is still a major cause of amputation despite the use of insulin, etc. Hopefully long-term treatment will progress and lessen the incidence from this cause.

Amputation for infection, such as osteomyelitis, tuberculosis and poliomyelitis, has been reduced by preventive medicine, and this trend can be expected to continue. The advances in the control of leprosy, tropical ulcers, etc., are reducing the incidence of amputation from these causes — another trend which can be expected to continue.

The advances in the understanding of the cause of neoplasia raise hopes that its incidence may be reduced by preventive measures.

ALTERNATIVE TREATMENT

Once a congenital skeletal defect occurs we cannot expect any major advance, except for the refinement of reconstructive surgery already used in the hand, and prosthetic replacement is likely to remain the solution.

The treatment of vascular disease, including diabetes, is improving both medicinally and surgically, and in the future many patients may be treated by these means, thus avoiding amputation altogether or at least employing a more distal amputation.

Infections have already been greatly reduced by antibiotics and other specific drugs, and this is a trend which must surely continue.

The advances in oncology are reducing the number of cancer patients who need amputation, and this is likely to continue. Even when surgical removal of a tumour becomes necessary there is the possibility of using an implanted skeletal prosthesis or a less radical amputation than hitherto.

PROSTHETIC REPLACEMENT

Changes in external limb prosthetics will depend upon new materials and new mechanisms being developed, after which new surgical techniques may be needed to take advantage of them.

Many new materials and new mechanisms have already been introduced into lower-limb prosthetics so that the single amputee can lead a satisfactory social life at any age with any level of amputation and have little restriction of occupation. A number of new devices are being developed which, when proven, will further improve the function of these prostheses, but major advances seem unlikely for some time to come.

Upper-limb prosthetics presents a different picture. Those currently available, complex as they may be, are still far from replacing the highly complex motor use of the upper limb, and give practically no sensory replacement. Furthermore, devices which provide some motor and sensory function detract from the appearance of the purely cosmetic replacement.

Upper limb

For sensory input the upper-limb amputee has had to rely in the past on sight and the reaction between the stump, socket and operating harness, together with sound. The use of external power increases the sensory deficit because it removes the operating controls from direct contact with the terminal device.

Research into providing sensory information additional to that already available is being pursued in many Centres, although it will be many years before a sensation remotely resembling the normal becomes available.

A kind of 'sensory' input has been devised which substitutes for those sub-critical reactions which are made without thought, in that a closed circuit can be designed which applies just enough grip to prevent slip, and responds automatically if, due to added forces, the object grasped begins to slip. This enables an egg to be held without either slipping or being crushed.

Systems giving a stimulus reaching a critical level have been tried in Japan, the USA, and elsewhere. They depend on transducers on the terminal device giving a quantitative but not qualitative stimulus to pressure, which is transmitted electrically to the body. It can then be used to stimulate a suitable sensitive area of skin which is not otherwise required for sensation or, as Clippinger of Duke University has shown, can stimulate a sensory nerve, via radio from an external antenna to an implanted receiver. The sensation provided is somewhat crude by either method and the techniques need refining, but this is a beginning of sensory prostheses in limbs.

It has been hoped that inert discs of carbon fibre, ceramic or other materials, which can be left in the skin without producing an inflammatory reaction, would allow prolonged penetration of the skin both for direct sensory input and motor controls. As yet a successful outcome seems to be remote although eventually it is hoped that this route may become practical. Indeed, it opens up possibilities of skeletal attachment in a more distant future.

External power has been in use for some time. Initially the external power source was either a pneumatic or electric motor, but the development of smaller, lighter, faster acting, and quieter electric motors and more durable, lighter, rechargeable batteries has made electric power the current choice. Lightness is a comparative term and as yet the motor, power-pack, and mechanism of the artificial hand are still heavy. They are placed in the prosthesis distal to the amputation stump and much of the energy, either of the patient or from the batteries, is employed in moving them rather than doing a useful 'pay-load'. Further reduction in size and weight is possible but one solution might be to have a more centrally mounted battery-pack and motor if a leakproof hydraulic system could be devised. This might provide a basis for

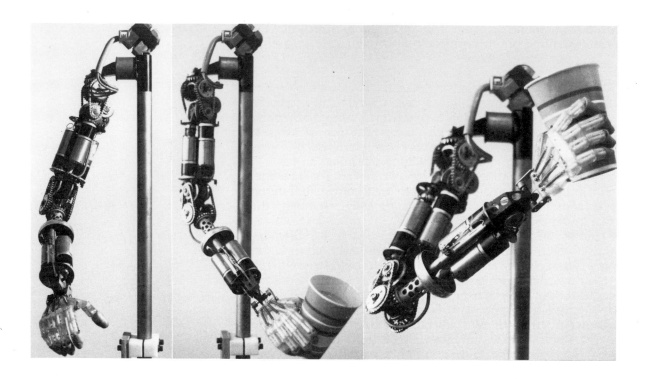

Fig. 17.1 An electrical robot arm utilizing a differential gearbox to enable natural arm movements to be carried out

multiple operation, which becomes more important in upper-arm amputations which require not only grip and rotation of the forearm, but also flexion and extension and rotation at the elbow.

Further development of control systems is needed, particularly in higher amputation, but unfortunately the higher the amputation the fewer the sites from which to gain control. Moss Rehabilitation produced a prototype using multiple myoelectric signals from the muscles of the shoulder girdle operating through a miniprocessor and using pattern recognition. Myoelectric is the current means of controlling the prosthesis, but there may be a return to mechanical controls in the future. Muscle bulge might return for use with some of the modern switch gear. At Johns Hopkins hospital, the attachment of cables to adhesions between underlying muscles and skin has been tried, and the introduction in the United Kingdom of the servo switch system, at present using conventional body power, offers the possibility of cineplasty. Unfortunately, although new materials have lightened the prosthesis, the armamentarium incorporated in them has, if anything, increased the weight.

Lower limb

The past decade has seen many improvements in lower-limb prostheses and there are many new devices in the prototype stage at the present time. Until recently prostheses had uniaxial joints giving movement in the sagittal plane, or sometimes had a single lateral ankle movement. It has long been recognized that normal gait had very considerable axial rotations in the various limb segments. This rotation was absorbed in the prosthesis by the superficial fascia of the stump. For many years flexible ankles were attempted, such as the US Navy ankle and the UK metalastic, but they were both heavy and lacked durability. Now it seems probable that a flexible ankle which is able to withstand the forces generated will be available shortly and there is now available a torque absorber or rotator positioned in the lower leg.

There are likely to be some further improvements on knee mechanisms but the major changes which will materially assist the amputee are in the use of lighter materials, such as carbon fibre, and compliant sockets.

Hitherto, although the overall length of the lower limb could be reproduced, the natural cadence of this compound pendulum could not be tuned to the other limb. Lightness in itself is not a virtue, for normal gait is in part dependent on decelerating the momentum imparted to the swinging limb. To lighten the limb for the elderly and feeble could only be done by lessening the proximal mechanisms and leaving the footwear, artificial foot and ankle the same, thus effectively lengthening the pendulum. The newer, lighter materials are now beginning to make it possible to tune the prosthesis to the natural cadence of the other limb, not necessarily by lightening it altogether but by adding some weight proximally.

The other major change which can be expected is the development of compliant sockets. The muscles of a stump contract and relax in active use and the stump therefore changes shape. Sockets must be rigid to transmit the forces developed. Hitherto sockets have largely been totally rigid and have therefore been compromises on the changing shapes of the stump. Lyquist of Copenhagen introduced an air-cushioned socket in 1968 for the patellar tendon prosthesis but it has not been widely used. Then recently, Wall in Sweden introduced a socket for the above-knee amputee which is rigid where required but allows the muscles to contract.

Eventually, when the mechanisms have been fully evaluated in the upper limb, it may be possible to use myoelectric controls for lower-limb mechanisms. However, the mechanisms now in use are coming closer to the natural action and by the time myoelectric controls are practical the mechanical devices are likely to be as good or superior.

Bibliography

Alter, A.H., Moshein, J., Elconin, D.B. et al (1978) Below knee amputation using the sagittal technique: a comparison with coronal amputation. *Clin. Orthop.*, **131**: 195–201.

Artificial Limbs. Published twice-yearly by the Committee on Prosthetic Research and Development and the Committee on Prosthetic/Orthotic Education of the National Academy of Sciences from 1954 to 1972. This journal contained high-quality articles on every aspect of the subject.

Batch, J.W., Splittler, A.W. & Metall, J.G. (1954) Advantages of knee disarticulation over amputation through the thigh. *J. Bone Jt Surg.*, **36A**: 921.

Blakeslee, B. (1963) *The Limb-deficient Child*. Berkeley, CA: University of California Press.

Bottomley, A.H. (1970) Control of the upper limb. In D.C. Simpson (ed), *Modern Trends in Biomechanics*. London: Butterworths.

Bremner, A.G. (1967) *Walking Skills for Amputees*. Auckland, NZ: Zealandia Catholic Newspaper.

Bulletin of Prosthetic Research. Published twice-yearly by the Prosthetic and Sensory Aids Service, Veterans Administration.

Burgess, E.M., Matsen, F.A., Wyss, C.R. et al. The below-knee amputation. *Interclin. Information Bull.*, **8**.(4): 1.

Burgess, E.M. & Matsen, F.A. (1981) Determining amputation levels in peripheral vascular disease. *J. Bone Jt. Surg.*, **63A** (9): 1493–97.

Burgess, E.M., Traub, J.E. & Wilson, A.B. (1967) *Immediate Post-surgical Prosthetics in the Management of Lower Extremity Amputees*. Washington, DC: Veterans Administration.

Burgess, E.M., Romano, R.L. & Zettl, J.H. (1969) *The Management of Lower Extremity Amputations*, 11 TR: 10–6. Prosthetic and Sensory Aids Service, US Veterans Administration.

Burgess, E.M. et al (1982) Segmental transcutaneous measurement of Po_2 in patients requiring amputation for peripheral vascular insufficiency. *J. Bone Jt Surg.*, **64A** (3): 378–82.

Coffman, D.J. (1979) Vasodilators in peripheral vascular disease. *N. Engl. J. Med.*, **300**: 715–17.

Crock, A.V. (1967) *The Blood Supply of the Lower Limb Bones in Man*. Edinburgh: Churchill Livingstone.

Dederich, R. (1963) Plastic treatment of the muscles and bone in amputation surgery. *J. Bone Jt Surg.*, **45B**: 60.

De Palma, A.F. (1964) *Clinical Orthopaedics and Related Research*, Vol. 37. Philadelphia: Lippincott.

Dewar, M.E., Coddington, T., Jarmon, P. et al. (1984) The role of thermography in the assessment of the ischaemic limb. In Ring, E.F.J. and Phillips, B. *Recent Advances in Medical Thermology*, pp. 345–50. London: Plenum Press.

DHSS Statistics and Research Division (1978) *Amputation Statistics for England, Wales and N. Ireland, 1978*. London: HMSO.

Dormandy, J. Peripheral ischaemia. *Viscositas*, V (**2–3**): 5–6.

Elert, C., Niebel, W., Karuse, E. et al (1976) The effect of Naftidrofuryl

(Praxilene) on energy metabolism in the musculature of limbs with impaired blood flow. *Therapiewoche*, **23**: 3947–50.

Engstrom, B. & Van de Ven, C. (1985) *Physiotherapy for Amputees: The Roehampton Approach*. Edinburgh: Churchill Livingstone.

Finch, D.R.A., Macdougal, M., Tibbs, D.J. et al. (1980) Amputation for vascular disease: the experience of a peripheral vascular unit. *Br. J. Surg.*, **67**, 233–37.

Fishman, S. Peizer, E., Kay, H.W. et al. (1962) *Metabolic Measures in the Evaluation of Prosthetic and Orthotic Devices,* New York University, NY: Research Division, College of Engineering.

Fulford, G.A. (1967) *Symposium on Amputation Surgery*. Queen Mary's Hospital, Roehampton.

Fulford, G.E. & Hall, M.J. (1968) *Amputations and Prostheses*. Bristol: John Wright.

Galvao, M.S. (1975) An improved technique for below-knee amputation. *J. cardiovasc. Surg.*, **16**: 603–8.

Gruss, J.D., Koradedos, C., Bortels, D. et al. (1981) Intra-arterial perfusion with prostaglandin E_1 for limb salvage in cases with severe inoperable occlusive disease. In *Hormones and Vascular Disease*, pp. 177–180. London: Pitman Medical.

Howard, P.R.S., Chamberlain, J. & Macpherson, A.I.S. (1969) Through-knee amputation in peripheral vascular disease. *Lancet*, **2**. 240.

Hunter-Craig, I., Vitali, M. & Robinson, K.P. (1970) Long posterior flap myoplastic below-knee amputation in vascular disease. *Br. J. Surg.*, **57**: 62–5.

Imperato, A M. Lumbar sympathectomy role in the treatment of occlusive arterial disease in the lower extremities. *Surg. Clin. N Am.*, **59** (4). 719–35.

Interclinic Information Bulletin. Published by Prosthetic and Orthotic Studies, New York University Medical School, and the Committee on Prosthetic Research, National Academy of Sciences.

Jain, K.J. (1982) *Transcutaneous oxygen tension measurement in the assessment of peripheral ischaemia in the lower limb*. M. Phil. thesis, University of Surrey. Department of Mechanical Engineering.

Jarrett, P.E.M. & Browse, N.L. (1981) *Anabolic Steroids and Vascular Disease*, pp. 190–196. London: Pitman Medical

Kendrick, R.R. (1956) Below-knee amputation in arteriosclerotic gangrene. *Br. J. Surg.*, **44**: 13–17.

Kihn, R.B., Warren, R. & Beebe, G.W. (1972) The geriatric amputee. *Ann. Surg.*, **176**: 305.

Klopsleg, P.E. & Wilson, P.D. (1959) *Human Limbs and their Substitutes*. New York: McGraw-Hill (reprinted 1968, New York: Hafner).

Little, J.M., Davis, B.C., Robinson, K.P. & Vitali, M. (1971) A pneumatic weight-bearing temporary prosthesis for below knee amputees. *Lancet*, **1**: 271–72.

McCarthy, G.T. (ed) (1984) In *The Physically Handicapped Child: An Interdisciplinary Approach to Management*, Chapter 11. London: Faber and Faber.

McCoullough, N. (1971) The dysvascular amputee. In *Current Problems in Surgery*. Chicago: Year Book Medical.

Ministry of Health (1967) *Immediate Post-operative Fitting*. London: HMSO.

Murdoch, G. (1968) Myoplastic technique. *Bull. pros. Res.*, Spring **10** (9): 4.

Negus, D. (1981) Prostacyclin and the ischaemic limb. In *Hormones and Vascular Disease*, pp. 181–89. London: Pitman Medical.

Parry, W (1981) Amputations of the upper limb. In *Rehabilitation of the Hand*, 4th edn. London: Butterworths.

Orthotics and Prosthetics. Published monthly by the American Orthotic and Prosthetic Association, Washington, DC.

Peizer, E. & Wright, D.W. (1970) Human Locomotion. In G. Murdoch (ed.) *Prosthetic and Orthotic Practice*, London: Edward Arnold.

Persson, B.M. (1974) Sagittal incision for below knee amputation in ischaemic gangrene. *J. Bone Jt Surg.*, **56B**: 110–14.

Prosthetics International. Published by the International Committee on Prosthetics and Orthotics of the International Society for the Rehabilitation of the Disabled, Copenhagen (no longer published).

Prosthetic and Sensory Aids Service (1969) *The Management of Lower Extremity Amputations*. Washington, DC: Veterans Administration.

Radcliffe, C.W. & Foort, J. (1961) *The Patellar-Tendon-Bearing Below-Knee Prosthesis*, pp 168–80. Berkeley, CA: University of California.

Redhead, R.G. & Snowdon, C. (1978) A new approach to the management of wounds of the extremities: Controlled environment treatment and its derivatives. *Prosth. Orth. Int.*, **2**: 148–56.

Redhead, R.G. et al. (1978) Post-amputation pneumatic walking aid. *Br. J. Surg.*, **65**: 511–12.

Robinson, K. (1980) Amputations in vascular disease. *Ann. R. Coll. Surg.*, **60**: 82–91.

Rose, G. (1981) Strategy of prevention: lessons from cardiovascular disease. *Br. Med. J.*, **65**: 267–71.

Royal College of Surgeons (1967) Report of a symposium on amputations and prosthetics held at the Royal College of Surgeons of England. *Ann. R. Coll. Surg.*, **40**: (4).

Simpson, D.C. & Kenworthy, G. (1973) Design of a complete arm prosthesis. *Biomed. Eng.*, **8**: 56.

Spence, V.A., Walker, W.F., Troup, I.M. and Murdoch, G. (1980) Amputation of the ischaemic limb; selection of the optimum site by thermography. *Angiology*, **32**(3): 155–69.

Swinyard, C.A. (1969) *Limb Development and Deformity: Problems of Evaluation and Rehabilitation*. Springfield, Ill.: Charles C. Thomas.

Termansen, N.B. (1977) Below knee amputation for ischaemic gangrene. Prospective randomised comparison of a transverse and sagittal operative technique. *Acta Orthop. Scand.*, **48**: 311–16.

Tracy, G.D. (1966) Below knee amputations of ischaemic gangrene. *Pract. Med. Surg.*, **74**: 251.

Wagner, F.W. (1977) Amputations of the foot and ankle: current status. *Clin. Orthop.*, **122**: 62–69.

Warren, R. & Kinn, R.B. (1968) A survey of lower extremity amputations for ischaemia. *Surgery*, (St Louis) **63**: 107.

Wilson, A.B. (1972) *Limb Prosthetics*. Huntingdon, NY: Robert E. Krieger.

Yao, S.T. & Irvine, W.T. (1969) Ankle systolic pressure measurements in arterial disease of the lower extremities. *Br. J. Surg.*, **56**: 676.

Index